HEALTH PROMOTION

Also by Angela Scriven:

Alliances in Health Promotion: Theory and Practice*

* Also published by Palgrave

Health Promotion

Professional Perspectives

2nd edition

edited by

Angela Scriven and Judy Orme

palgrave in association with The Open University

First published 2001 by
PALGRAVE
Houndmills, Basingstoke, Hampshire RG21 6XS and
175 Fifth Avenue, New York, N.Y. 10010
Companies and representatives throughout the world

PALGRAVE is the new global academic imprint of
St. Martin's Press LLC Scholarly and Reference Division and
Palgrave Publishers Ltd (formerly Macmillan Press Ltd).

ISBN-13: 978-0-333-94834-7 paperback
ISBN-10: 0-333-94834-3 paperback

This book is printed on paper suitable for recycling and made from fully managed and sustained forest sources.

A catalogue record for this book is available from the British Library.

Editing and origination by
Aardvark Editorial, Mendham, Suffolk

10 9   8   7
10 09 08 07 06 05

Printed and bound in Great Britain by
Creative Print & Design (Wales), Ebbw Vale

Contents

List of Figures and Tables

Figures

Tables

Notes on Contributors

Lee Adams has worked for 25 years in the Health Service in Health Promotion. She is currently the Director of the Health Action Zone for Wakefield District and is also a member of the UKPHA (UK Public Health Association) Council. She is author of numerous publications.

Peter Allen is Head of Environmental Health at Oxford City Council and a Member of Green College, Oxford. He has written and lectured extensively on health promotion in local government.

Yvonne Anderson is a senior manager in the NHS and visiting fellow at the University of Southampton. She formerly worked with a range of voluntary organisations, at both a local and national level, in both a paid and unpaid capacity.

Alan Beattie's career as a practitioner and researcher in health promotion spans 20 years in the NHS, school and voluntary settings, as well as universities. Alan was involved in the development of health promotion courses and research projects at London University from 1977 to 1989. He has been Honorary Senior Research Fellow in Applied Social Science at Lancaster University since 1989 and is currently Professor of Health Promotion.

Norma Daykin is Head of the School of Health Sciences in the Faculty of Health and Social Care at Glenside at UWE, Bristol. She has taught the sociology of health and illness course for 10 years, during which time she has also researched and published in a range of health-related areas. In 1999 she co-edited, with Professor Lesley Doyal, *Health and Work: Critical Perspectives*, (Macmillan).

Mark Dooris is a Senior Lecturer in Health Studies at the University of Central Lancashire in Preston, where he also coordinates the Health-promoting University initiative. He has previously worked in a range of roles within local authority and health service settings, has carried out consultancy work for the WHO Regional Office for Europe and has written extensively on settings-based health promotion and sustainable development.

Stephen Farrow is a Public Health Professor at Middlesex University and a Director of Public Health in Barnet. Previous posts include Director of a University Institute that specialised in the evaluation of healthcare. He has worked extensively on a range of projects and has acted as a consultant for the World Health Organization, as well as many other national and international organisations.

Robin Ireland formed Healthstart in 1995 after 13 years of promoting physical activity and a healthier lifestyle. Healthstart organises events and campaigns with a health message, but with the emphasis on having fun as you become fitter. The service provided for the NHS in the North West received a National Beacon Award for health improvement in 1999. Healthstart specialises in health at work and green transport programmes.

Linda Jones is Senior Lecturer in Health and Well-being in the School of Health and Social Welfare at the Open University and has chaired and contributed to many of its health courses. Her research interests focus on policy change in health promotion and public health, and, in particular, on the role of transport in determining access and independence for vulnerable groups.

Sue Latter is Reader in Nursing at the University of Southampton. She has experience as a nurse in both hospital and community settings, and has subsequently focused on researching and teaching health education and health promotion with undergraduate and postgraduate healthcare professionals. Her research interests and publications have focused on the application of health education and health promotion within nurse education and practice, including establishing the evidence base for effective interactions, and patient/user involvement in healthcare and healthcare research.

Alyson Learmonth has over 20 years' experience as a health promotion specialist. She is currently Health Promotion Strategist for County Durham and Darlington Health Authority and English Chair of the Society of Health Education and Promotion Specialists. Her areas of interest include primary care, evidence-based practice, mental health promotion and addressing inequalities in health.

Jennifer Lisle has a broad professional background in public health, psychological medicine and occupational health. As Director of Joint Research and Health Advisers since 1985, she has worked with both public and private sectors on a wide range of organisational health issues. She is a Senior Visiting Fellow at the Institute of Health Sciences, City University, London.

Sally Markwell is the Coordinator for the Health for All partnership with Winchester City Council and has worked within the public health sector for over 20 years. She also worked for nine years in Eastern Europe as a volunteer, researching and developing health education and promotion in Romania, Serbia and Kosovo. She has developed multi-sectoral partnerships within local government and health sectors across England and Wales, and has most recently been an advisor for the WHO/EURO Verona Initiative for Investment for Health, with direct involvement in the production of the Verona Benchmark.

Kate Marsden is the Consumer Relations Officer at University Hospital Queens Medical Centre NHS Trust in Nottingham. As part of the Quality and Consumer Relations team, Kate has been involved in running focus groups related to patients' complaints and their impact on practice, and with issues surrounding the development of patient participation. She was a contributing editor to *Self Help: An Annotated Bibliography 1983–1993*, published by Self Help Nottingham.

Tom Mellish is Health and Safety Policy Officer at the TUC, where he has worked for over 11 years. His work involves research and policy development on a wide range of health and safety at work issues, including EC health and safety directives and their implementation in the UK. His remit also includes psychosocial issues such as alcohol and drugs in the workplace, stress and bullying, and he is author of the TUC guide *Tackling Stress at Work* as well as co-author of the TUC's *No Excuse – Beat Bullying at Work*.

Jan Myers lectures part time at Nottingham Business School, Nottingham Trent University, where she is also undertaking part-time research. She continues to work in the voluntary sector on organisation development and health issues such as community involvement in Health Action Zone initiatives, in primary care and on a freelance consultancy basis with voluntary and public sector organisations. From 1996 to 1999 she was director of Self Help Nottingham. In 1998 she co-authored *Self Help Groups: Getting Started, Keeping Going* and contributed to *Living with the Legacy of Abuse* (Engel) with a chapter 'Self Help Groups for Partners'.

Judy Orme is a Principal Lecturer in Health Promotion at the University of the West of England in Bristol. She has been working in this field for more than 20 years and has published widely. Her research interests include the sociology of public health, young people and drug-taking behaviour and primary care development.

Sue Robertson is a Senior Lecturer in Community and Youth Work at the University of the West of England in Bristol. She has over 20 years' experience in the Youth Service as a youth worker and manager in a variety of different settings and areas.

Wendy Rose is a Senior Research Fellow of the School of Health and Social Welfare at the Open University. She was formerly Assistant Chief Inspector (Children's Services) in the Department of Health. She has recently been developing, with the Department of Health, a framework for assessing children in need and their families.

Angela Scriven is the Award Leader for Professional Health Programmes, including the MSc in Health Promotion, at Bath Spa University College. She has been teaching in this field for over 20 years and has published widely. Her research is centred on the relationship between health promotion policy and practice within specific contexts. She is the editor of *Health Promotion Alliance: Theory and Practice*.

Viv Speller is Executive Director of Health Improvement at the Health Development Agency. Her background is in psychology and behavioural studies, and she has worked in the field of health promotion in Manchester, London, Hampshire and Wessex. She was Senior Lecturer in Health Promotion at the University of Southampton and retains research links with its School of Nursing and Midwifery.

Jane Thompson is a Senior Lecturer in Health Studies at St Martin's College, Carlisle. She has a background as a health promotion specialist and is currently involved in teaching and research. Her current research interests include sexual health and young people, and sustainable community and health development.

Keith Tones is a Senior Associate Lecturer at the Nuffield Institute, Leeds and was Professor of Health Education at Leeds Metropolitan University until retiring a few years ago. He has been involved in postgraduate health education teaching for over 20 years and has acted as a consultant for the World Health Organization and many other international and national organisations. He has published extensively on health education, promotion and public health, and is also Editor of the international journal *Health Education Research*.

Gill Velleman is the Chief Officer for South East Bristol Primary Care Group. Prior to this, she worked in health promotion for 12 years and managed Health Promotion Service Avon. She is interested in developing evidence-based healthcare and has significant experience of planning and organising health programmes.

Elizabeth Williams is the Programme Manager for South East Bristol Primary Care Group, with responsibility for implementing the Health Improvement Programme. She worked as a teacher, and was then a health promotion specialist for 14 years. During this period, she was acting head of a growing health promotion department with a remit for planning and managing health promotion. In 1999 she moved from the Health Promotion Service to become Programme Manager at South East Bristol Primary Care Group.

Cheryl Wright is an experienced nursing professional with a background in midwifery and health visiting, in addition to six years' experience as a senior manager with responsibility for a range of community nursing disciplines. She is currently working in a dual role between the Bath and West Community as a Community Health Manager and Bath Spa University College as a Senior Lecturer Practitioner.

Acknowledgements

We would like to thank all of the contributors to this second edition and those who helped with the development of ideas in individual chapters.

Special thanks to Tracey Awramenko for her support during the early preparation of the manuscript and to April Setchfield for her diligence, patience and sense of humour when supporting the finalising of the manuscript.

Every effort has been made to trace all the copyright holders but if any have been inadvertently overlooked the publishers will be pleased to make the necessary arrangements at the first opportunity.

List of Acronyms

AA	Alcoholics Anonymous
AMMA	Assessment Masters and Mistresses Association
CPHVA	Community Practitioners and Health Visitors Association
DCMS	Department for Culture, Media and Sport
DES	Department of Education and Science
DETR	Department for the Environment, Transport and the Regions
DfEE	Department for Education and Employment
DoE	Department of the Environment
DoH	Department of Health
DoT	Department of Transport
EC	European Commission
EHO	Environmental Health Officer
ENHPS	European Network of Health-promoting Schools
GEST	Grant for Education Support and Training
GMB	General, Municipal and Boilermakers Union
GMS	Grant-maintained school
GP	General Practitioner
HA	Health Authority
HAZ(s)	Health Action Zone(s)
HEA	Health Education Authority
HEBS	Health Education Board, Scotland
HImP	Health Improvement Programme
HLC	Healthy Living Centre
HSC	Health and Safety Committee
HSE	Health and Safety Executive
ILO	International Labour Organisation

INSET	In-service training
ITT	Initial teacher training
LA	Local Authority
LGA	Local Government Association
LGMB	Local Government Management Board
LMS	Local management of schools
NCC	National Curriculum Council
NCVO	National Council for Voluntary Organisations
NFER	National Foundation for Educational Research
NHS	National Health Service
OHS	Occupational Health Service
PCG	Primary Care Group
PCT	Primary Care Trust
PGEA	Post Graduate Education Award
PHC	Primary healthcare
PSHE	Personal, social and health education
QCA	Qualifications and Curriculum Authority
RCN	Royal College of Nursing
SEU	Social Exclusion Unit
SHEG	Scottish Health Education Group
SHEPS	Society for Health Education and Promotion Specialists
SMEs	Small enterprises
TUC	Trades Union Congress
UKCC	United Kingdom Central Council for Nursing, Midwifery and Health Visiting
UKPHA	UK Public Health Association
WHO	World Health Organization

Introduction

ANGELA SCRIVEN AND JUDY ORME

Health promotion has evolved into an extremely broad sphere of activity encompassing health education, lifestyle and preventative approaches alongside environmental, legal, policy and fiscal measures designed to advance health. Given this comprehensive range of approaches, it is not unexpected that, in addition to the key functions of professionals working in specialist units, the promotion of health has an established position in the remit of a variety of professional groups. The publication in 1996 of the first edition of *Health Promotion: Professional Perspectives* was welcomed by health professionals and academics alike because it was the first book to identify and concentrate specifically on the diversity of professional groups who have an interest in and a responsibility for health promotion. The second edition of this text has the same aim as the first, which is to provide a concise, accessible and up-to-date account of the diversity of professional practice in promoting health. More specifically, individual chapters will explore how professional domains and organisational and policy contexts can influence the range and nature of interventions.

The Health of the Nation (DoH, 1992) dominated the chapters in the first edition, but *Saving Lives: Our Healthier Nation* (DoH, 1999) has superseded this strategy. The revised edition reflects this and the wide range of other policy changes that have occurred in the five years since the first publication. Professionals now operate in organisational environments dominated by policy themes (such as social inclusion) that have emerged from what the current Labour government has termed 'the third way'. *Saving Lives: Our Healthier Nation* reflects this third-way political movement by putting on to the new public health agenda the objective of redressing inequalities. To counter the possibility of being accused of political rhetoric, a range of strategies, such as Health Action Zones, have been put in place that are intended to achieve this objective. These strategies will be considered in some detail in the various chapters in this text.

In a similar way to its predecessor, *Our Healthier Nation* calls for the establishment of collaborative partnerships between the various agencies and professional groups that promote health. Multiprofessional collaborative partnerships are now seen as an important prerequisite to achieving the new public health targets. They are part of the other policy themes that have emerged in the three years since the Labour government came to office, such as 'joined-up thinking' and 'seamless care', which, when applied across government departments, should avoid the introduction of contradictory policies. Establishing these collaborative partnerships requires careful consid-

eration. There is a need for constructive communication and a full understanding of the structure, philosophy, constraints on and possibilities for
health promotion in a range of professional spheres of work.

There are a number of inherent difficulties associated with the promotion
of health through collaborative partnerships. The success of interagency
health promotion initiatives is dependent on numerous factors. A key issue is
undoubtedly the different interpretations and ideological understanding of
health promotion that the various agencies and their respective professional
representatives espouse. Approaches that encompass the full range of para-
digms and are underpinned by a clear understanding of the principles of
health promotion might require some professional groups to make uncomfortable shifts in ideology.

Another tension is that collaborative partnerships are often advocated as a
cost-effective way of providing health promotion, in that the outcome is
hoped to be more than the sum of the parts. However, funding considerations sometimes militate against such partnerships, as will become evident in
some of the chapters that follow. Uncertainties surrounding future organisational structures and financial arrangements often oppose the formation of
effective partnerships. The level of policy and related organisational change
since the last edition of this book will undeniably have resulted in some
modified professional remits, organisational restructuring and changes to
funding arrangements.

The central purpose of this second edition is to offer an extensive insight
into the variety of professional perspectives on health promotion. It is
intended as a text that might increase understanding and thus facilitate the
process of joint working between professionals drawn from different backgrounds with different cultures and ideologies. Because of its approach, the
book will appeal to a wide range of readers including the following specialist
groups and students training to become members of these groups: health
promotion specialists, nurses and health visitors, professions allied to medicine such as physiotherapists, social workers, teachers/lecturers/trainers,
local edcation authority health education coordinators/advisers, environmental health officers and specialists in public health medicine.

There are a distinguished group of academics and health professionals who
have contributed to this second edition, many of whom have revised their
chapters from the first edition. The list of more than 20 authors includes
representatives from specialist health promotion, health services, local
authorities, voluntary organisations and the education sector. New chapters
highlight some of the recent significant changes in the National Health
Service (NHS). The emerging role of Primary Care Groups (PCGs) and
Primary Care Trusts (PCTs) in health promotion will be covered in a chapter
written by two new contributors, both of whom are actively engaged in the
management and research of a PCG. A new chapter on the enhanced role of
community nurses covers policy initiatives such as Health Improvement
Programmes, Health Action Zones and Healthy Living Centres. Other new

contributors provide a chapter on health promotion in higher education, drawing on examples from the health-promoting university project and assessing the changing role of national agencies in influencing professional perspectives and partnerships.

The same six parts as were in the first edition are used to structure the text. These sections continue to reflect the professional settings within which health promoters operate. As with the first edition, however, the settings are not seen as exclusive or definitive; it is recognised that some professionals work across professional boundaries and settings. For the purposes of this book, for example, the chapter on school nurses will again appear in the education and youth setting even though they are, as a professional group, employed by the health service. Additionally, education has not been incorporated into the local authority setting. The contributions within the education and youth setting are much wider than local authority statutory education provision. A new feature of the second edition is an introduction at the beginning of each part that will offer an overview identifying the key issues and provide an additional stimulus for debate.

Part I is the portion of the book that deals with a number of issues of relevance to the consideration of health promotion in different professional settings. Keith Tones begins with an updated analysis of the concept of health promotion and the importance of the synergistic relationship between significant approaches.

The efficacy of working across professional boundaries receives special attention from Sally Markwell and Viv Speller in Chapter 2. These new contributors deal with the conceptual basis of interprofessional collaboration and offer an overview of the potential and pitfalls of partnership work across professional boundaries in the context of current policies, including the Verona Initiative. These two chapters, forming the first part of the book, establish the issues, dilemmas and debates that will permeate the chapters that follow.

Part II of the book focuses on the health service, contributions reflecting the wide range of professional activities that are a key feature of health promotion practice within this sector. The section begins with Lee Adam's overview of the implications for health promotion of the recent NHS reorganisation. The focus on health authorities provides a critical assessment of the constraints and opportunities for health promotion in the wake of the NHS reforms.

Gill Velleman and Elizabeth Williams add to this debate by providing an analysis of the emerging role of the PCGs and PCTs. The pivotal role of these agencies in facilitating health promotion work is highlighted, and the autonomy that these bodies have to develop their own priority areas is assessed.

Cheryl Wright follows this by considering the enhanced role of community nurses in the delivery of health promotion in community settings. Policy initiatives such as Health Improvement Programmes, Health Action Zones and Healthy Living Centres are explored in some depth in this chapter.

Alyson Learmonth then provides a critical evaluation of the recent changes within the specialist health promotion service.

Sue Latter concludes Part II by revising her detailed exploration of the opportunities available for health promotion in hospital nursing practice. The nurses' specific role as health educators with patients is reviewed, followed by a critical analysis of nurses' potential for collaborative health promotion partnerships. Constraints that may militate against the achievement of this potential are highlighted.

Part III includes three chapters concentrating on the health promotion work of local authorities. Contributions centre on the development of health promotion within this sector at both local and national levels.

Peter Allen initiates this debate with an evaluation of the extent to which environmental health services engage in health-promoting activities and an assessment of how the discretionary powers of environmental health officers can be used to this end.

Following on from this, Linda Jones and Wendy Rose evaluate the potential for promoting health in the very pressured realm of social service provision. The barriers of a defensive culture will be taken into account, and links will be made with all aspects of social service provision. The potential for collaborative work between social services and health services is explored in some detail.

Robin Ireland examines the connections between sport and health by considering the roles of the Sports Council, national agencies and local authorities. The potential for partnerships between local authorities, health services and the community is explored, and issues relating to participation in sport and the role for health promotion are discussed.

Part IV is concerned with the range of health promoters who operate within the education and youth work professional domain. Angela Scriven assesses the issues concerned with the delivery of health education in schools. The discussion on the impact of government education policy will focus on health education within the National Curriculum framework, the role of local education authorities and the position of health education in initial teacher training. Alan Beattie follows this with a revised analysis of the health-promoting school initiative, applying models or frameworks of health promotion.

The opportunities and strengths of the school nurse as a health promotion agent are examined by Stephen Farrow. The vulnerability of this particular group of health promoters is discussed in some detail. Jane Thompson and Mark Dooris' new chapter draws on their involvement in the Health-promoting Universities project and will discuss the potential for health promotion in the non-statutory education sector. Sue Robertson concludes this section by assessing the potential within youth settings for health promotion. Examples of good practice are highlighted.

Part V focuses on voluntary organisations. Yvonne Anderson will provide a new overview of the opportunities for health promotion within this setting.

The impact of recent legislation, organisational structures and funding pressures will be given prominence as important considerations for health promoters. Jan Myers and Kate Marsden address the concept of self-help and critically examine the role of self-help groups in promoting health.

Part VI considers health promotion within the workplace. The opening chapter by Norma Daykin explores the context of workplace health promotion, tracing the link between health and work and examining the various levels of intervention for promoting the well-being of people in the workplace. Tom Mellish examines the important role of the trade unions in promoting health. The underlying premise here is that the place of trade unions is as a part of any process involving decisions that will affect the health and well-being of employees.

The final chapter of the book is written by Jennifer Lisle, who focuses on the role of the occupational health services, exploring opportunities for health promotion in the context of organisational structure. Her analysis centres on the need for these services to adopt a proactive role in developing appropriate organisational strategies to support healthy organisations.

Finally, each chapter uses the current policy contexts to explore the implications for practice for the professionals working in a range of environments. It is intended that this second edition will provide new and important insights into the possibilities and constraints when implementing the diverse range of initiatives and activities that take place under the auspices of health promotion.

References

Department of Health (1992) *The Health of the Nation*. London: HMSO.
Department of Health (1999) *Saving Lives: Our Healthier Nation*. London: HMSO.

PART I

ISSUES CONCERNED WITH THEORY AND PRACTICE

INTRODUCED AND EDITED BY ANGELA SCRIVEN

Part I of this book examines issues surrounding theory and practice in health promotion, and as such is intended to introduce a range of ideas and arguments that create a context for what follows in the remaining sections.

Tones, in the first chapter, opens with a wide-ranging discussion of the concept of health promotion. While recognising that any analysis of the meaning of health promotion has traditionally resulted in dispute, Tones offers us a contentious view, describing health promotion as a militant wing of public health. In doing this, he presents his own well-established formula for health promotion, which is a combination of healthy public policy and health education. His justification for this explanation involves taking the reader on a potted history of the international policies that have shaped the development of health promotion to its current position. His assessment of empowerment is detailed and enlightening, making a strong case for moving beyond an ideological commitment to a technology incorporated seamlessly into health promotion work.

There are clearly issues in this chapter that have resonance in other parts of the book, such as the voluntary sector elements, Anderson in Chapter 16 presenting a case for the participative nature of voluntary services, reflecting the more empowering models of health promotion. Moreover, the section on the education and youth work setting, which offers an assessment of the health-promoting school and the new National Curriculum guidelines for personal and social education, reflects the action competencies and empowerment debates presented by Tones.

Marwell and Speller continue the discourse around recent developments in health promotion, with a particular emphasis on policy relating to partnership working. This chapter provides an important backdrop to the specific chapters on professional settings that follow. The various policy documents that give direction to the wide range of current initiatives that come under the aegis of health promotion are identified, outlined and evaluated. The authors present the background to the current position in which individuals, groups and organisations are not only encouraged, but also expected to work in collaborative ways to achieve goals outlined in the new public health

1

agenda. The difficulties and pitfalls of engaging in collaborative partnerships are examined in some depth. The impression given is that there is still much to do to overcome these difficulties, including the development of programmes of education and training that facilitate new ways of working that will harmonise and integrate health promotion activities across professional and organisational boundaries. The new Verona Initiative is outlined and clearly offers exciting opportunities for improving the quality and scope of partnership working. Overall, Tones and Marwell and Speller provide excellent insights into the range of debates that permeate the current environment in which health promoters operate. These chapters form a necessary framework from which to study the professional perspectives that are the focus of this book.

CHAPTER 1

Health Promotion: The Empowerment Imperative

KEITH TONES

This chapter will briefly review the essentially contested concept of health promotion and examine the formulation that the World Health Organization (WHO) has developed, largely since the launch of the movement to achieve Health for All by the Year 2000 (HFA2000) at the 30th World Health Assembly in 1977. More particularly, it will consider the empowerment imperative contained within this formulation and provide an ideological model of health promotion based on the assertion that health promotion's primary concern should be with helping people to gain control over their lives and their health. An examination of both community empowerment and self-empowerment will be followed by a brief reference to the ways in which these principles might be applied to health promotion settings and methods.

The meaning of health promotion

Health promotion is an essentially contested concept: it is used in a variety of ways by different individuals and organisations, typically in the context of special pleading or in support of some cherished viewpoint or philosophy. It is not uncommon to consider health promotion as being synonymous with health education, or to view health education as part of health promotion. The term 'health development' is, on occasion, used as being equivalent to health promotion, and recently the concept of health promotion has been seen to differ little from that of public health. Indeed, health promotion is sometimes considered to be part of public health or, conversely, public health is sometimes viewed as a component of health promotion. Over 10 years ago, Green and Raeburn (1988: 30) provided a rather appropriate description of the ways in which various individuals and groups made their bids for ownership:

> Ideologues, professionals, interest groups, and representatives of numerous disciplines have attempted to appropriate the field for themselves. Health and education

professionals, behavioural and social scientists, holistic health and self-care advocates, liberals, conservatives, voluntary associations, funding agencies, governments, community groups, and many others all want something from health promotion, all want to contribute something, and all bring their own orientation to bear on it.

In order to avoid further ideological argument, health promotion will, for the purpose of this chapter, be considered to be a kind of militant wing of public health. Its essential components are twofold and give rise to the following formula:

Health Promotion = Healthy Public Policy × Health Education

The term 'healthy public policy' is borrowed from the Ottawa Charter, its major purpose being to create legislation, economic and fiscal measures and various forms of social and environmental engineering in order to make the healthy choice the easy choice. Without appropriate health policy, health education will in many instances be unable to influence healthy choices. On the other hand, without health education, it will frequently be impossible to develop and implement healthy public policy, especially those policies which are politically problematic. Health education is readily defined as follows:

> Health education is any intentional activity which is designed to achieve health or illness related learning, i.e. some relatively permanent change in an individual's capability or disposition. Effective health education may, thus, produce changes in knowledge and understanding or ways of thinking; it may influence or clarify values; it may bring about some shift in belief or attitude; it may facilitate the acquisition of skills; it may even effect changes in behaviour or lifestyle. (Tones and Tilford, 1994: 11)

In the model of health promotion proposed below, the purpose of healthy public policy and health education should be to empower individuals and communities, and reduce or remove the various barriers preventing the attainment of health for all.

A comprehensive account of health promotion and its history is beyond the scope of this chapter, and more complete analyses may be found elsewhere (see, for example, Anderson, 1984; Tones, 1985; Minkler, 1989). However, since the empowerment imperative is central to the WHO's conviction about the purpose of health promotion and its definition, the following important milestones marking progress from the 1977 initiation of HFA2000 will be briefly noted.

Milestones in health promotion

At one level, it could be argued that the roots of health promotion are to be found in the WHO's original and classic definition of health (WHO, 1946), with its holistic emphasis on well-being. It is, on the other hand, important also to note the change of emphasis embedded in HFA2000: health is no longer viewed as the ultimate purpose of health promotion but instead a means to an end, namely the attainment of a socially and economically productive life. This clearly begs the question of the nature of social and economic productivity, but it is nonetheless a rather more manageable concept than perfect well-being!

The most obvious precursor to health promotion is undoubtedly the Declaration of Alma Ata (WHO, 1978), which, *inter alia*, asserted that the existence of gross inequalities between advantaged and disadvantaged peoples was politically, socially and economically unacceptable. The proposed solution to this problem was to be Primary Healthcare (PHC). This is not to be confused with primary *medical* care since *demedicalisation* was to be an important thrust of PHC and, subsequently, health promotion. Moreover, given the perspective of the present book, we should also acknowledge how Alma Ata popularised the notion of intersectoral collaboration.

If Alma Ata and PHC were the prototypes, the emergence of health promotion as a major movement was formalised with the publication by WHO's European Region of its concepts and principles in 1984. Kickbusch (1986: 438) described this event as 'a new forcefield for health [which] integrates social action, health advocacy and public policy'. The first full blossoming of the principles incorporated in the 1984 publication was arguably to take place in Ottawa, when 200 delegates from 38 nations made a commitment to health promotion in what has, since that time, been celebrated as the Ottawa Charter (Kickbusch, 1986; WHO, 1986).

The specific features of the Charter may be consulted elsewhere, and its principles will feature in the more extended review that is presented below. It is, however, worth noting that although reference was made to the importance of developing people's personal skills, health education was dislodged from the centre-stage position it enjoyed under the aegis of PHC and was virtually replaced by the enthusiasm for building healthy public policy. As we will note later, this was a fundamental flaw. The other most important ideological principle to emerge from Ottawa was its reiteration that the empowerment of individuals and communities should be a major focus of future work: community action must be strengthened and decision making facilitated by creating supportive environments. The theme of demedicalisation was also maintained and found expression in the argument for the reorientation of health services in order to both expand their scope and make them more user friendly.

Health promotion's progress was maintained by both attempts to activate the 38 targets for achieving HFA2000 (WHO, 1985) and a number of subsequent conferences and major initiatives. A second international conference on health promotion was, for example, held in Adelaide (Green and Raeburn, 1988) which pursued ways of building healthy public policy, and, most recently, a third international conference was held in Sundsvall (WHO, 1991). The Sundsvall Declaration focused on the need to provide supportive environments for health and highlighted four aspects: the social dimension, the impact of cultural norms and social processes; the political dimension, the requirement on governments to guarantee democratic participation in decision making and make a commitment to human rights and peace; the economic dimension, the need to re-channel resources to achieve health for all; and finally, the need to recognise women's skills and knowledge.

In addition to the conferences and declarations, attempts to translate rhetoric into practice are especially relevant to the aims of this book. The most significant of these was perhaps the Healthy Cities movement, which initially sought to establish test beds for health promotion in 11 European cities. A more extended discussion of Healthy Cities may be consulted elsewhere (see, for example, Fryer, 1988 and Kickbusch, 1989). Suffice it to say that this WHO-inspired development acted as a stimulus for the emergence of more than 300 local initiatives in various European cities. In addition to the focus on the city, the principles of health promotion were applied to a number of more specific institutions, organisations and contexts, a development that has become widely known as the Settings Approach.

The most recent and important of WHO's milestones has been the Jakarta Conference (WHO, 1997, 1998). In short, the Jakarta Declaration reiterated the importance of the Ottawa Charter principles.

Ottawa: key principles

WHO has consistently advocated a positive and holistic view of health and asserted that it comprises mental, physical and social elements rather than merely being concerned with the prevention and control of disease. In addition, Ottawa and Jakarta have identified the following major concerns for health promotion:

- *Equity.* The ultimate concern of health promotion lies with the achievement of equity and social justice; avoidable inequalities in health between and within nations are intrinsically unacceptable. Equity is not only a worthwhile goal in its own right but a means to the end of preventing disease and premature death.

- *Empowerment.* Helping people to gain control over their lives is both a prime goal in its own right as well as the major means of achieving equity. In order to achieve this goal, a supportive environment must be created at all levels. This will be achieved in two main ways:

- building healthy public policy to address the major determinants of health and illness that reside in the physical, cultural and socio-economic environment in which people live and work;
- strengthening individuals' personal competencies and capacities.

- The achievement of active participating communities.

- *The reorientation of the health services.* Health is too important to be left to the medical profession: there must be a reorientation and reframing of health services. Since medical services often do not meet population needs and can be disempowering, they should be reformed. Demedicalisation is an important goal of health promotion. Not only is it concerned with shifting the balance of power from doctors and the medical establishment towards patients and clients, but it also seeks to acknowledge the substantial contributions made by other services to health and illness. Services such as housing, transport, leisure and recreation, and economic development, may all influence health for good or ill. Since so many organisations, contexts, settings and services can influence health, collaborative working is, by definition, likely to maximise their impact. Intersectoral collaboration is therefore a key instrumental principle for maximising the health-promoting potential of these services and for influencing the development and implementation of healthy public policy.

Health promotion, empowerment and reciprocal determinism

The concept of empowerment is complex and, as with health promotion, comprises an amalgam of ideological and technical attributes. A full discussion is not therefore possible here, and a more complete analysis may be found elsewhere (Tones, 1992, 1994, 1998a; Tones and Tilford, 1994). Figure 1.1 seeks to demonstrate the relationship between health promotion, empowerment and the attainment of health.

In the last analysis, the concept of *reciprocal determinism* (Bandura, 1982, 1986) lies at the very heart of the empowerment imperative in health promotion. Reciprocal determinism is one of the central tenets of social learning theory and asserts that people's capacity for action, and ultimately their health, is determined by the nature of their environment. On the other hand, however, it is usually possible for people to exercise at least some degree of control over their circumstances. The relationship between environment and individual is thus one of reciprocity, except for those individuals who are continually overwhelmed by so many negative events and oppressive circumstances that their degree of choice is effectively zero.

As noted earlier, health is ultimately determined by the existence of equity and social justice, and this is in turn rooted in people's material, social, economic and cultural circumstances. Following the Ottawa mandate, the

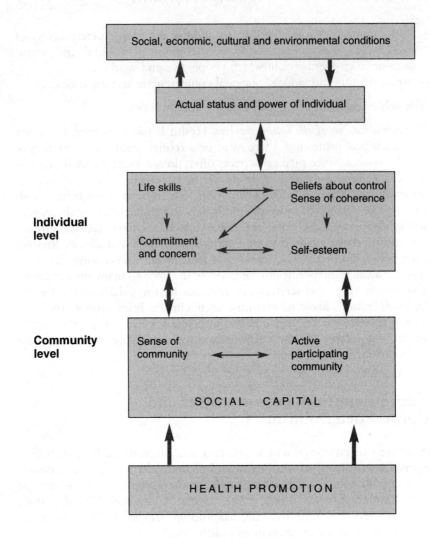

Figure 1.1   The reciprocal influence of empowerment and the environment

creation of healthy public policy is the prerequisite for changing adverse environments in order to facilitate the achievement of health. Empowerment best describes how the barriers to implementing healthy public policy might be overcome.

In short, two interrelated forms of empowerment ultimately contribute to the achievement of health status; these are individual empowerment and community empowerment. Community empowerment is most readily characterised by the terminology of the Ottawa Charter as an active participating community. Individual empowerment, or self-empowerment, might be defined as follows:

> Empowerment is a state in which an individual actually possesses a relatively high degree of power: that is having the resources which enable that individual to make genuinely free choices. Power cannot be absolute – and even if it could, it would be undesirable since it would militate against the right of other people to make choices. Indeed, one of the key features of empowerment is that system of checks and balances which safeguards the rights of others.
>
> Individual empowerment is associated with certain beneficial psychological characteristics of which the most significant are: beliefs about personal control – including realistic causal attributions – together with a relatively high level of self esteem based on a realistic self concept; valuing other people and their rights to self determination; possession of a repertoire of health and life skills. (Tones, 1994: 169)

Figure 1.1 shows a reciprocal relationship between community empowerment and individual empowerment. This relationship is based on the premise that an active, participating community to some extent comprises the sum of empowered individuals within that community. Certainly, empowered individuals are needed to mobilise communities in their quest to challenge adverse circumstances. On the other hand, an empowered community will also generate norms and a social support system that will reinforce individual empowerment, and individuals within an empowered community are more likely to acquire the competencies and characteristics that lead to self-empowerment.

Figure 1.1 also shows two related features of empowered individuals and communities. The first of these is a *sense of community*, a state characterised by four key dimensions:

- membership – a feeling of belonging;
- shared emotional connection – the commitment and belief that members have shared and will share history, common places, time together, and similar experiences;
- influence – a sense of mattering;
- integration and fulfilment of needs – a feeling that members' needs will be met by the resources received through their membership in the group. (McMillan and Chavis, 1986: 9, cited from Tones, 1998b: 189)

We might note here that aspects of this sense of community and, indeed, the notion of an empowered community in general are closely related to the currently popular formulation of *social capital* (Putnam et al., 1993), a desirable state in its own right and a state that is considered to be health promoting and, at the same time, conducive to self-empowerment for its members.

In Figure 1.1, individual empowerment has been associated with *sense of coherence*. This term was coined by Antonovsky (1979: 123), who defines it as:

> a global orientation that expresses the extent to which one has a pervasive, enduring though dynamic feeling of confidence that one's internal and external environments are predictable and that there is a high probability that things will work out as well as can reasonably be expected.

While both a sense of community and a sense of coherence are related to empowerment, it is important to strike a cautionary note. Antonovsky uses the term 'negentropic' when describing the results of a sense of coherence. In other words, a sense of coherence militates against the perception of life in general. A sense of coherence, on the other hand, creates the impression that life is comprehensible: the world is ordered, consistent, structured and clear, and the future predictable.

However, while an empowered individual or community is likely to hold such views, it is possible also to conceive of individuals and communities who are not empowered also holding such beliefs! It is possible, for example, for oppressed masses to believe that their dreadful circumstances are the will of God (who, of course, moves in mysterious ways but tends to offer the tanta-lising prospect of future rewards in some better place); to quote Voltaire's Doctor Pangloss, 'All is for the best in the best of possible worlds.' Marxists make a similar point in their reference to the concept of *false consciousness*. As we will note below, health promotion must be concerned with achieving social and political change; a sense of community and a sense of coherence must also be challenged where these are based on false consciousness.

The dynamics of self-empowerment

Figure 1.2 shows the relationship between some of the factors traditionally associated with the state of self-empowerment.

The reciprocal relationship between environment and individual is again prominently displayed. Beliefs about control are central to the empowered state, and the conviction that people are in charge of their destiny *in general* has been consistently associated with empowerment. This personality trait, associated with Rotter's (1966) well-known construct of *perceived locus of control* has been extensively researched and associated, with several beneficial health outcomes.

The concept of self-efficacy (Bandura, 1982) is, however, more useful in devising health promotion programmes for individuals. In short, apart from acquiring an appropriate knowledge and understanding of the implications of health actions and having a positive attitude to the relevant health-related behaviours, people must actually believe that they are capable of carrying out those health actions. The best way to influence self-efficacy beliefs is of course

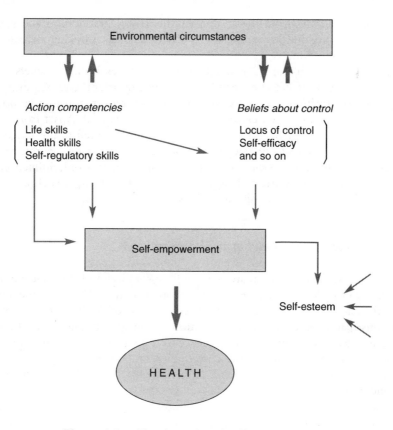

Figure 1.2   The dynamics of self-empowerment

to provide individuals with experience of success (the second-best procedure being to provide them with credible models who have already experienced success and with whom they can identify).

A prerequisite for success is the provision of training for the acquisition of essential skills, described here generically as *action competencies*. In Figure 1.2, action competencies are subdivided into three categories of skill. The first of these is labelled life skills and refers to general capabilities that can enhance people's success and survival in everyday living. Life skills typically include a number of key social interaction skills in addition to specific psychomotor skills that might be needed, for example, to adopt a safe and effective exercise regime. Some of the more frequently described life skills have to do with relaxation, time management and assertiveness.

The term 'health skill' has been employed where the skills are associated with achieving preventative outcomes. Self-regulatory skills, on the other hand, relate to the long-established tradition of behaviour modification. This has been increasingly exploited to help people to control difficult decisions and the negative effects resulting from them, typically the loss of gratification and gain in discomfort from quitting unhealthy practices such as smoking or excessive alcohol consumption.

The resulting mix of skills and beliefs contributes both to beliefs about being in control of life and health and, more importantly, to acquiring the actual power to influence one's environment. Moreover, through empowerment, the individual's self-esteem is likely to be enhanced. Apart from being an important mental health goal in its own right, a realistically based and relatively high level of self-esteem is associated with making healthy choices in general. Figure 1.2 reminds us that self-esteem is not only influenced by empowerment, but is affected by a number of other factors, such as feeling respected and loved by significant others.

An empowerment model of health promotion

Figure 1.3 seeks to encapsulate the key philosophical and strategic elements of the health promotion enterprise envisioned by the WHO and the author of this chapter. It is based on the interpretation of health promotion as a synergistic interaction of health education and healthy public policy. In addition to generally demonstrating the centrality of education, it shows the ways in which individual and community empowerment influences the social, economic and environmental determinants of health through healthy public policy.

The Ottawa Charter emphasised the importance of *lobbying, advocacy and mediation* in achieving healthy public policy. Lobbying is a well understood procedure and needs no further explanation here. Advocacy is the form of lobbying that occurs when relatively powerful individuals or agencies act to produce change on behalf of those lacking in such power, such as dispossessed communities or patients experiencing the often intimidating encounter with doctors.

The Ottawa Charter recognised that there was often, and perhaps inevitably, a conflict of interest between health promotion policies and other political imperatives concerned with, for example, fostering economic growth. Accordingly, mediation between conflicting interests was an important aspect of the process of policy development. The importance of intersectoral collaboration at the macro level is also acknowledged in Figure 1.3 by demonstrating the influence of 'coalitions' of the 'great and the good' and the powerful on the policy creation process.

Reference was made earlier to the need not only to reorient the health services to make them more accessible and user friendly but also to broaden the definition of the ways in which services other than medical services contribute to health. Accordingly, the health policy is necessary in order not only to reorient but also to reframe the perception of health services.

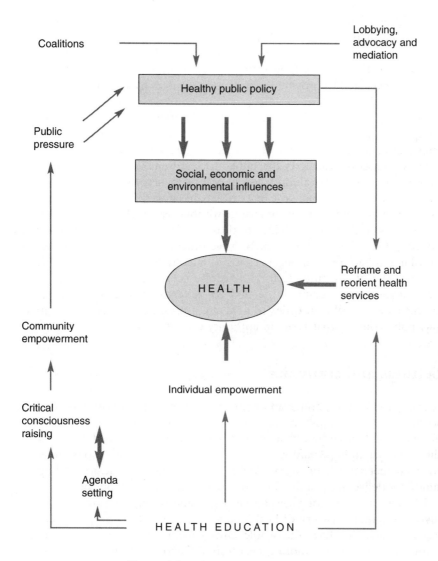

Figure 1.3　An empowerment model
(adapted from Tones and Tilford, 2001)

The contribution of health education cannot be overestimated; it involves a focus on the individual, a focus on the community and a focus on the health services. The individual focus differs dramatically from health education's traditional and often 'victim-blaming' stance. Instead of seeking to persuade people to adopt preventative behaviours and *comply* with the prescriptions of health professionals, the aim is to empower by strengthening individual capabilities, as detailed above, and facilitating choice of action.

Health education still has a part to play in working with health services, but rather than persuading individuals to make appropriate use of those health services, it instead seeks to alert decision makers to the health promotion role of the services they manage. Again, health promotion specialists might be expected to provide training and resources to assist with tasks associated with that role.

Most importantly of all, however, health education has a critically important and radical function that can be encapsulated in the notion of community empowerment. At one level, it is charged with agenda setting. This is defined here as a process that alerts the public to important but politically sensitive health issues such as the fluoridation of water supplies. Its purpose is primarily to create a climate of opinion that will enable government, for example, to institute and claim the credit for change without risking electoral unpopularity.

Much more difficult to tackle are those fundamental health issues such as poverty and disadvantage which governments and other agencies are unwilling to address, either because of ideological conviction or, again, through fear of courting electoral disaster. Accordingly, the strategy of critical consciousness raising is needed to generate public indignation and concern about health in order to generate a pressure for change, or preferably public outcry, that those in authority cannot resist.

Settings and strategies

A discussion of the settings and contexts of health promotion is beyond the scope of this chapter and will receive further attention in the rest of this book. We will merely note here that the settings approach developed by the WHO differs in certain important respects from earlier conceptualisations, especially the view that schools or the workplace, for example, provide an ideal opportunity for delivering health education to an often captive population.

In short, the current view is that a genuine settings approach does not involve the mere delivery of health education but instead adopts an ecological approach in which the whole environment and ethos of a particular setting is geared to promoting health in a coherent and integrated fashion. Furthermore, a health-promoting setting should relate in a collaborative manner to the community in which it is situated.

The empowerment initiative is, of course, central to the settings approach and various specific empowering strategies might well be used within different contexts. Three of these will now be briefly summarised below:

- *Media advocacy*. The most important role for the mass media is in the support of interpersonal initiatives and, above all, in raising critical consciousness about health issues generally, a process now typically described as media advocacy. For a more complete discussion of this, see Tones (1996a) and Chapman and Lupton (1994).

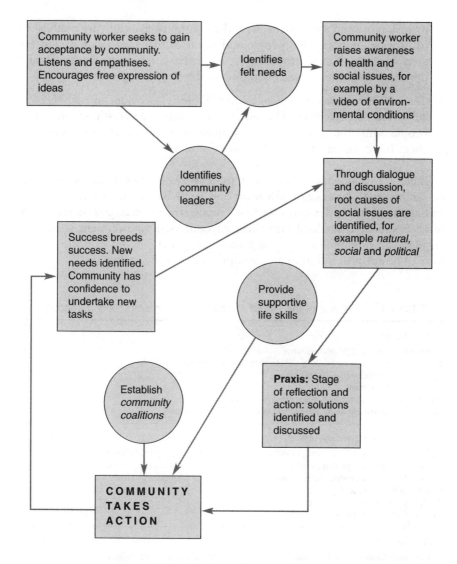

Figure 1.4   Praxis and community action

- *Community development and critical consciousness raising.* Figure 1.4 summarises the key processes involved in a community empowerment approach operating within a community development context.

    Figure 1.4 (Tones, 1996b) incorporates Freire's (1972) recommendations on what is sometimes called emancipatory education. This is a dialectical process that involves critical consciousness raising, subsequently leading to praxis, that is, the translation of critical thinking about social issues into action. Freirean dialectics are, however, supplemented by the provision of supportive life skills, and community coalitions are established to provide support from people and agencies that exercise power in the given setting. The empowering role of the community worker/health promoter is consistent with community development practice.

● *The empowering face-to-face encounter.* Table 1.1 provides an analysis of an empowering encounter. The one-to-one encounter clearly involves two people. Only the task of the health professional is shown; the task of the client has been omitted for the sake of simplicity.

Table 1.1 is intended to remind us that face-to-face work is the most common health promotion situation and is to be found in virtually every setting. It seeks to demonstrate that empowerment strategies at the micro level should be embedded into these encounters. Empowerment is not just an ideological commitment: it is a technology that should be incorporated into all health promotion in an appropriate but seamless fashion.

Table 1.1   The role of the health professional in an empowering encounter

---

Communication

Check felt needs/need for information
Establish rapport using counselling skills: active listening and so on
Take account of non-verbal messages
Check for understanding
Check intelligibility of any written information provided
Take steps to maximise recall and provide aide-memoire if necessary

---

Motivation: facilitating decision making

Explore existing beliefs, attitudes and skills; seek to modify beliefs, especially beliefs about control. Explore attitudes and underlying values
Provide information; provide skills: decision making, psychomotor, social and life skills
Check learning and recall
Analyse environmental circumstances
Negotiate and agree 'contract'

Provide support

Provide opportunity for acquiring supportive knowledge and social and self-regulatory skills
Help mobilise social and environmental support
Act as advocate for social and environmental change
Check client's progress

References

Anderson, R. (1984) Health promotion: an overview. In Baric, L. (ed.) *European Monographs in Health Education Research*, No. 6. Edinburgh: Scottish Health Education Group.
Antonovsky, A. (1979) *Health, Stress and Coping*. San Francisco: Jossey-Bass.

Bandura, A. (1982) Self-efficacy mechanism in human agency. *American Psychologist*, **37**(2): 122–47.

Bandura, A. (1986) *Social Foundations of Thought and Action: A Social Cognitive Theory*. New Jersey: Prentice Hall.

Chapman, S. and Lupton, D. (1994) *The Fight for Public Health: Principles and Practice of Media Advocacy*. London: BMJ Publications.

Freire, P. (1972) *Pedagogy of the Oppressed*. Harmondsworth: Penguin.

Fryer, P. (1988) A healthy city strategy three years on – the case of Oxford City Council. *Health Promotion*, **3**(2): 213–18.

Green, L.W. and Raeburn, J.M. (1988) Health promotion. What is it ? What will it become? *Health Promotion*, **3**(2): 183–6.

Kickbusch, I. (1986) Issues in health promotion. *Health Promotion*, **1**(4): 437–42.

Kickbusch, I. (1989) Healthy cities: a working project and a growing movement. *Health Promotion*, **4**(2): 77–82.

McMillan, D.W. and Chavis, D.M. (1986) Sense of community: a definition and theory. *Journal of Community Psychology*, **14**: 6–23.

Minkler, M. (1989) Health education, health promotion and the open society: an historical perspective. *Health Education Quarterly*, **16**: 17–30.

Putnam, R.D., Leonardi, R. and Nanetti, R.Y. (1993) *Making Democracy Work: Civic Traditions in Modern Italy*. Princeton, NJ: Princeton University Press.

Rotter, J.B. (1966) Generalised expectancies for internal versus external control of reinforcement. *Psychological Monographs*, **80**(1): 1–28.

Tones, B.K. (1985) Health promotion: a new panacea? *Journal of the Institute of Health Education*, **23**: 16–21.

Tones, B.K. (1992) Health promotion, empowerment and the concept of control. In Colquhoun, D. (ed.) *Health Education: Politics and Practice*. Victoria, Australia: Deakin University Press.

Tones, B.K. (1994) Health promotion, empowerment and action competence. In Jensen, B. and Schnack, K. (eds) *Action and Action Competences*. Copenhagen: Royal Danish School of Educational Studies.

Tones, B.K. (1996a) Models of mass media: hypodermic, aerosol or agent provocateur? *Drugs: Education, Prevention and Policy*, **3**: 29–37.

Tones, B.K. (1996b) Health education, behaviour change and the public health. In Dettels, R. and McEwen, J. (eds) *Oxford Textbook of Public Health*. Oxford: Oxford University Press.

Tones, B.K. (1998a) Health education and the promotion of health: seeking wisely to empower. In Kendall, S. (ed.) *Health and Empowerment: Research and Practice*. London: Edward Arnold.

Tones, B.K. (1998b) Empowerment for health: the challenge. In Kendall, S. (ed.) *Health and Empowerment: Research and Practice*. London: Edward Arnold.

Tones, B.K. (2001) Health promotion, health education and the public health. In Dettels, F., McEwen, J., Bealehole, R. and Tanaka, H. (eds) *Oxford Textbook of Public Health* (4th edn). Oxford: Oxford University Press (in press).

Tones, B.K. and Tilford, S. (1994) *Health Education: Effectiveness, Efficiency and Equity*. London: Chapman & Hall.

Tones, B.K. and Tilford, S. (2001) *Health Promotion: Effectiveness, Efficiency and Equity* (3rd edn). London: Stanley Thornes (in press).

World Health Organization (1946) *Constitution*. Geneva: WHO.

World Health Organization (1978) *Report on the International Conference on Primary Health Care, Alma Ata, 6–12 September*. Geneva: WHO.

World Health Organization (1984) *Health Promotion: A Discussion Document on the Concept and Principles.* Copenhagen: WHO.

World Health Organization (1985) *Targets for Health for All.* Copenhagen: WHO.

World Health Organization (1986) *Ottawa Charter for Health Promotion: An International Conference on Health Promotion, November 17–21.* Copenhagen: WHO.

World Health Organization (1991) *Sundsvall Statement on Supportive Environments for Health, 9–15 June.* Geneva: WHO.

World Health Organization (1997) *The Jakarta Declaration on Leading Health into the 21st Century.* Geneva: WHO.

World Health Organization (1998) *New Players for a New Era: Leading Health Promotion into the 21st Century. 4th International Conference on Health Promotion, Jakarta, Indonesia 21–25 July, 1997.* Geneva: WHO.

CHAPTER 2

Partnership Working and Interprofessional Collaboration: Policy and Practice

SALLY MARKWELL AND VIV SPELLER

There have in recent years been profound changes in the policies relating to partnership working and interprofessional collaboration for the development of the public health workforce in order to improve the delivery of public health and health promotion actions. Changes in practice have followed, initially piecemeal, with little development and support, but progressing to substantial shifts in working practice with calls for systematic development and training. This chapter charts the changes in policy in partnership working and public health development, highlighting some of the achievements, difficulties and needs for future development.

Partnership working

The major changes that have taken place in health promotion since the Ottawa Charter were acknowledged in the Jakarta Declaration of 1997 (WHO, 1998a: 7). Clear evidence was put forward that comprehensive approaches to health development are most effective, the Jakarta Declaration calling for an increased investment in health, the empowerment of individuals and the public, increased social responsibility for health and the consolidation of the infrastructure of health promotion.

World Health Organization (WHO) strategies for dealing with equity and healthcare have emphasised the need for an intersectoral approach to health (WHO, 1997), identified the value of intersectoral action for poverty reduction and promoted the need for stronger partnerships for health between the private and public sectors and civil society (WHO, 1998b).

Over the past 10 years, UK government policies have begun to redirect their efforts towards supporting health strategies that encourage individuals, groups and organisations to work together through recognising the common ground between them and agreeing on shared objectives (DoH, 1993). Collaborative alliances have emerged from the public sector arena in response to *Health for All by the Year 2000* (WHO, 1988) and subsequently the government's health strategy *The Health of the Nation* (DoH, 1992), which has been recognised as the driving force behind the early interest of the National Health Service (NHS) in, and support for, the development of healthy alliances (Speller, 1998).

With the election of a new government in the UK in 1997 and the appointment of a Minister for Public Health, health promotion was due to have a much higher profile. With the promise of action to tackle inequalities and the encouragement of more healthy partnerships between councils and health authorities, the development of partnerships was seen to be crucial (Chambers, 1997).

A range of modernising initiatives has emerged, aimed at facilitating closer working between local agencies and thus providing the means to work together with other independent bodies, as well as local communities and individuals, to pursue joint objectives (DoH, 1999a). In the NHS, these ideas are now firmly rooted within the policy outlined in the White Paper *The New NHS: Modern, Dependable* (DoH, 1997a). A third way of running the NHS is proposed as a system based on partnership and driven by performance. Health Improvement Programmes (HImPs) set the framework for the services that NHS Trusts provide and the detailed agreements they make with Primary Care Groups. The duty of partnerships also required participation alongside universities and local authorities (NHS Executive, 1999). The vision for the future of social services emphasised greater joint working between social services, health and housing, as well as the use of pooled budgets (DoH, 1998a). The developments in access to funding (underpinning joint working approaches, including joint appointments, pooled budgets and joint investments plans) were introduced in the *Partnership in Action* discussion document (DoH, 1998c). In addition, the New Opportunities Fund, set up in 1998, emphasises the cross-over between traditional local authority areas, such as education and social services, to focus on the broader determinants of ill health and the development of community-based Healthy Living Centres (New Opportunities Fund, 1999).

Plans for the future of local government continued this theme of joint working by setting out a vision of councils listening to the people they serve, building up their communities, working in partnership with others and delivering efficient services to high standards (HMSO, 1998). Local authorities have a new duty to take a lead role in promoting the social, economic and environmental well-being of their communities through the development of a community plan, setting the broad objectives or vision for a local community (DETR, 1999). Social inclusion is currently one of the most active stimuli for partnership working, identified within the Crime and Disorder Act of 1998. It places new obligations on agencies and local authorities to work together in partnership to develop and implement a strategy to reduce and tackle crime and disorder in their areas. A significant development in community justice is the emergence from within communities of a partnership approach between interested groups and agencies, supported by statutory bodies such as the police and the probation services (Newell, 2000). The recognition of the need to produce 'joined-up solutions' to 'joined-up problems' was emphasised in the creation of the Social Exclusion Unit in 1997 to improve government action to reduce social exclusion (SEU, 1998).

The White Paper relating to education, *Excellence in Schools* (DfEE, 1997), proposed that schools should become healthy workplaces for staff and children. The paper reflects the commitment of the government, through the Department of Health and the Department for Education and Employment, to work in partnership with the private and voluntary sectors, local agencies and the communities they serve to build sustainable healthy schools (DfEE, 1997). This has been consolidated in the development of the National Healthy Schools Standard, which requires local healthy schools programmes to work in partnership at a strategic and operational level (DfEE, 1999).

The Green Paper *Our Healthier Nation* (DoH, 1998b) set out proposals for concerted action by the government, both as a whole and in partnership with local organisations and communities, to improve people's living conditions and health. Health authorities were given the key role in developing HImPs to identify local needs and translate the national contract into local action, local authorities working in partnership with the NHS to plan for health improvement.

Following widespread consultation, the third White Paper, *Saving Lives – Our Healthier Nation* (DoH, 1999b), sets out the strategic priorities for health over the next 10 years. It emphasises how new mechanisms, such as Health Action Zones, together with community plans, will become a key part of the delivery system for the achievements of the health strategy. The paper identifies the importance of intervening in social, economic and environmental areas to secure better health. It also recognises that people can make individual decisions about their own and their family's health, and presents an action plan to tackle poor health by improving the health of everyone, especially the worst off. The key to health improvement throughout this document is a new balance in which people, communities and government work together in partnership:

> the key to success is joint working at every level. This means that central Government departments must work with the health and local authorities, voluntary organisations, community groups and the private sector... we and all these agencies must involve the public in making decisions that are going to affect them. (DoH, 1997b)

In Scotland, the Green Paper on public health recognised the task of building a healthier Scotland as one that needed the formation of strong partnerships between local authorities, voluntary organisations, the private sector and the health service, and that these should reach out into local communities and involve the public in their activities (Scottish Office/DoH, 1998).

Working Together for a Healthier Scotland emphasises the need to address the health inequalities between Scotland's well-off and deprived communities and sets out measures to tackle ill health through local government functions such as education, housing and community care.

Similar approaches have been taken in Wales, where, building on existing health gain targets, there is a commitment to developing additional indicators relating to inequalities and health determinants (Welsh Office, 1998a). The establishment of the National Assembly with devolved responsibility for policies and standards of public services has been a significant change. Partnership is a key theme for the Assembly and is identified as a core value underpinning *Better Health, Better Wales* (Stationery Office, 1998a). The framework for partnership in policy development at various levels has been strengthened in a number of ways. The Assembly has developed a compact with both the voluntary sector and local government. A Partnership Council enables Assembly members and local government members to discuss issues of concern. To take partnership working between local government and the NHS a step further, the Health Act 1999 introduces new flexibility for joint working and the pooling of budgets, along with a duty of cooperation between NHS bodies and local government (Perry and Markwell, 2000).

Concerns have, however, been raised over the failure of *Saving Lives* (DoH, 1999b) to analyse properly the public health contribution of local authorities and the non-government sector, which appears to be subordinate to that of the NHS (LGA, 2000). The issues include the need for explicit guidance on the links between local authority community plans and HImPs, and further development of the public health role of local authorities in the wake of the new power to promote the social economic and environmental well-being of local communities. It has been argued that agencies at national, regional and local levels need to address public health issues in their policies and activities, and, most critically, to ensure that improving health and regenerating local communities are seen as mainstream issues for local government (LGA, 2000).

One of the recommendations of the Hunt Committee in its report *Rebuilding Trust* (House of Lords, 1995–96) was that local government should be encouraged to develop its role as the community leader, best able to take an overall view and to determine priorities. It is hoped that, under a revision of particular Sections of the Local Government Act 1972 relating to cooperation and partnership, joint arrangements with other statutory bodies may be established to pool or share resources and delegate responsibility for decisions within an agreed framework (DETR, 1999). *Modernising Local Government* (DETR, 1998) reiterates the Government's pledge to modernise the country and to bring the government back to the people. Local government has a key role to play in improving people's quality of life, which may be achieved through councils gaining a new democratic legitimacy, following new ways of working and adopting new disciplines such as best value.

As local authorities are increasingly seeing their role as one of community governance and community leadership, councils are being described as:

> moving away from the traditional narrow concept of partnership to a model that is broader and which embraces some very non-traditional working styles and relationships. This brings the realisation that the partnership culture requires new ways of working and new perceptions on roles and responsibility. (Improvement and Development Agency, 2000: 62)

This recognition that partnership working requires particular attitudes and skills is only now beginning to gain prominence, although there were earlier attempts to develop approaches to partnership working. This is addressed in the second part of this chapter, which looks at needs and difficulties, and sets the development of partnership-working skills in the broad context of the public health development agenda in the UK.

Public health development and interprofessional collaboration

The Chief Medical Officer's project to *Strengthen the Public Health Function in England* (DoH, 1998d) recognises the public health function in its widest sense, rather than just the contribution made by public health professionals, and the need for these to work collaboratively: 'if practitioners from different backgrounds do not work effectively together, opportunities will be lost – this will be particularly important for all those involved in public health' (DoH, 1998d: 4). This engagement of the wider public health workforce was signalled in *Saving Lives*, public health development work has proliferated at regional and national levels, and will be consolidated in the development of a Public Health Workforce Development Plan. Standards for public health for the UK are being developed under the auspices of the Tripartite Group, formed in 1998 from the Royal Institute of Public Health and Hygiene, the Multidisciplinary Public Health Forum and the Faculty of Public Health Medicine.

The Health Development Agency was formed in 2000 as a special health authority in England. Its remit was to improve health and reduce inequality in health by developing and maintaining an evidence base of effective action, which turned the evidence base into effective practice by building up the skills and capacity of the public health workforce, and advised on the setting of standards for public health planning and practice. In 2000, it will report on the development of methodology and the initial findings from an audit of public health skills. Thus, the definitions of core competencies and skills, as well as the strategic approach to implementing these through public health development programmes at regional level, are now being firmly established (see, for example, NHS Executive, 2000).

Within these approaches, skills of working across professional boundaries and within partnerships are clearly identified as prerequisites for effective practice. It is, however, important to recognise that these are not synonymous. A study of interprofessional education and training needs in public health in the South West of England drew distinctions between multiprofessional education and interprofessional education and learning, the latter being defined as a process in which different professions learn from and about each other in order to develop collaborative practice (CAIPE, 1994; Royle et al., 1999). Thus, interprofessional learning provides a foundation for partnership-working, while within the skills necessary for effective public health practice, particular attention needs to be paid to partnership working. In this survey of practitioners, over half identified the need to develop their partnership working skills and the need for closer working with other sectors for their jobs in the future (Royle et al., 1999).

While these initiatives demonstrate a clear commitment to development in these areas, earlier work has called for partnership development and identified specific prerequisites drawn from practice that will need attention (Powell, 1992; DoH, 1993; Markwell, 1994; Funnell et al., 1995). For example, key ingredients recognised by councillors as being necessary for successful working include creating a partnership agenda, building community capacity and focusing on partnership achievement (Improvement and Development Agency, 2000). The guidance also identifies a wide range of skills required by local councillors involved in developing and sustaining partnership working: facilitating discussion between partners, listening, building consensus, probing partners, a commitment to providing resources, building trust, enabling and empowering others, joint decision making, conflict handling and influencing skills. Recognising the contribution of workers in sectors outside the NHS will be fundamental to achieving the public health development goals outlined above, but infrastructural and resource issues are likely to continue to be an impediment for some time to come.

Since the early 1980s, many local authorities have begun to re-examine their potential role in promoting the public health, drawing in part on initiatives such as Health for All 2000 and Healthy Cities. When *The Health of the Nation* (DoH, 1992) was published, it attracted considerable criticism from local authorities. The narrow focus on disease models and measurable disease reduction targets, the neglect of key socio-economic and environmental determinants of health and the allocation of lead responsibilities for the national strategy within health were not easily reconciled with rhetoric about healthy alliances and little commitment to significant new resources. A study of the role of local authorities in promoting community health focused upon process issues of joint working relationships, working with the community and promoting quality of life (Speller, 1999). Respondents reported enthusiasm in their concern for and consideration of the factors that promoted health in their communities but frustration in their attempts to take action through resource limitations, lack of political support and difficulty in working across agencies. In relation to joint working in particular, there was a desire for a pragmatic approach to partnership work:

> The great successes in achieving good collaboration and community engagement were thought to be tangible projects with visible outcomes. There was a very clear understanding that developing alliances took time and considerable effort; and the experience of many was that it brought considerable benefits but that much remained to be done. (Speller, 1999: 63)

The need for health alliance work to be part of the statutory functions of the local authority was repeatedly mentioned, the role of Health for All coordinators being seen to be vital 'because they are trying to be a bridge between a number of organisations' (Speller, 1999: 48). Social capital building appeared to be as relevant for the community of agencies working in partnership as for the wider community. 'Effective partnerships were built on trust, expectation reciprocity of actions and strong networks of contact and information sharing. Where there were deficits in these, partnerships were less effective or had broken down' (Speller, 1999: 65).

Piloting of the National Occupational Standards for Professional Activity in Health Promotion and Care included testing in the local authority setting, drawing on the experience of workers based in local authorities with a broad responsibility for developing and coordinating partnerships for health promotion (HEA, 1998). Their roles, identified at the interface between organisations, were in general jointly funded, their main remit being to develop and sustain the work of health alliances in their local authority locality.

Specific aspects of the work of 'Health for all coordinators' was identified during the piloting which discusses the level of facilitation as well as operational management that the coordinator roles involved. In particular the roles were described as being part of a process of bringing people together, and keeping them together, requiring the ability to build relationships between individuals and agencies, having good communication skills, an ability to work collaboratively, and being able to negotiate a path often through many different agendas.

The National Occupational Standards for Professional Activity in Health Promotion and Care were derived from the job competence model, which acknowledges the complexity of work activity and the contribution of various types of knowledge and experience to successful performance. This model includes crucial aspects of competence:

- *task management*: the skills necessary to coordinate and manage the job role;
- *task skills*: the skills to do the job;
- *environmental management*: the awareness and management of the effect of external issues;
- *contingency management*: the ability to manage variance and contingency.

A further assessment of health alliance activity in the UK has been undertaken, involving a purposive sample of alliance facilitators attending the Health for All Network's national conference in 1997 (Markwell, forthcoming). Surveys were distributed among the group, which aimed to identify the general structures and functions of alliances, common barriers and outcomes of working plus potential training needs. Survey questions were drawn from sources of theoretical perspectives regarding organisational development (Handy, 1995), project management (University of Reading, 1994a), group processes (Huczynski and Buchanan, 1991; Douglas, 1995), conflict management (Sampson and Marthas, 1981), enabling structures (University of Reading, 1994b), process indicators of alliance working and basic descriptions of alliance formation (Funnell et al., 1995). Professional development for alliance leaders/facilitators tended to be fairly restricted, with a preponderance of support for information technology. Development needs and preferred training areas expressed by facilitators tended to fall within the frameworks of management development, alliance and community development, as well as theoretical approaches concerning health promotion.

Projects and their successful management have become a favourite instrument in recent years for performing new and highly complex tasks in organisations or in the cooperation between organisations, but projects are effective only when they are carefully and properly managed. Working in projects provides great opportunities for developing professional roles and sometimes establishing new ones. A project has been defined by Grossman and Scala (1993: 56) as 'a form of organisation to cope with complex, new, risky, intersectoral tasks within and between organisations, and an instrument of planned organisational change'. While the success of a project is determined by the quality of the project's content and the acceptance of the proposal by the people concerned, projects can develop their innovative function only by developing an autonomous activity on the one hand while maintaining and using their connections to the parent organisation(s) on the other.

Understanding the disadvantages and pitfalls of working together across agency and professional boundaries is further discussed through illustrations of a range of alliance structures and the explication of appropriate evaluative processes in Scriven (1998). The recognition of the barriers of working across intersectoral boundaries (Delaney 1994, 1996), the difficulties of the organisation in participating in partnerships while experiencing change (Speller, 1999), and the clear links identified between conflict, change and organisational development (Markwell, 1998) have certainly been highlighted over the past five years. These add to our understanding of the ability of partnerships to become agents for change, and of the professional development required in order to maximise their impact on health. More recently, work using the alliance evaluation framework (Funnell et al., 1995) in Wales has demonstrated how the process of collaborative audit of alliance function, combined with development activities, can contribute to alliance performance (Speller et al., 2000).

The process of devising monitoring and evaluation tools, and the use of those measures to review the progress of the alliance activities and development, has had two benefits. The first is the obvious one of measuring aspects of its work, but it has also provided an insight into issues within the fabric of the partnership that might need addressing in order to strengthen the potential for health improvement. At this point, it has served to strengthen the common understanding of a broad definition of health as well as to improve communication and therefore relationships. It has caused the partnership to prioritise areas of weakness, or opportunity, including a better representation of partner agencies, the profile and identity of the alliance, a knowledge of its potential, or even existence, in some sectors, and its links to developing policy and other influential groups.

This approach of audit and review in order to develop practice is enshrined in the new policy agenda of Best Value in local government (Welsh Office, 1998b; DETR, 1999), which aims to provide a more collaborative approach to improving standards of public service. Best value, as set out in the Local Government Act 1999, is defined as a duty to deliver services to clear standards, covering both cost and quality, by the most economic, efficient and effective means possible. Best value requires local authorities to ask themselves fundamental questions about the underlying objectives and priorities of their work and about their performance in relation to that of other organisations in the public, private and voluntary sectors. The government will also work with local government, in particular with the Local Government Association and the new Improvement and Development Agency, to help to manage, motivate and facilitate change. A beacon scheme aiming to modernise local government has now been introduced and will be a key element of this. The scheme will have two phases: the first phase will focus on spreading best practice; the second will, in addition, allow new freedoms and flexibilities to be tested (DETR, 2000a). In year two, the second phase, themes for Beacon Council Status 1999/2000, partnership may be found as a key element in measuring the impact of local work in the areas of community safety, education, health and supporting independent living for older people (DETR, 2000b).

Beacon status is, however, only part of the picture. Best value pilots, the Local Government Improvement Model and the work of the Improvement and Development Agency will all contribute. Further initiatives will be taken as the framework for modernisation is put in place to help councils to introduce best value, the new political structures and the new ethical framework (DETR, 2000a).

The recognition that the promotion of health needs to be addressed by concerted strategic action on the part of all levels and sectors of society has been formalised by the WHO in the development of the Verona Initiative Investment for Health approach (Ziglio et al., 2000). This has led to the development of the Verona Benchmark, a partnership benchmarking tool derived from benchmarking processes for business excellence in the private sector. Building on the work of the Verona Initiative and experience in good practice in partnership working, the tool allows for the individual and collaborative assessment of key partnership processes and outputs. It has been tested in a number of pilot sites in cities and areas in Europe, and has been found to be useful for partnerships in various stages of development towards an investment for health approach (Haglund et al., 2000; Perry and Markwell, 2000; Watson et al., 2000).

In this first piloting phase, it is clear that experienced facilitation to support the benchmarking process and to draw out the lessons for development, the sharing of ideas and experiences across partnerships and opportunities for education and training support in areas identified as needing further development are all required. A second phase of piloting is planned in 2000–01 with revised tools, and it is hoped that this will give a clearer indication of learning needs to direct educational programmes of relevant national agencies. The new public health agenda will require the harmonisation and integration of efforts to improve health and society, and to reduce inequality in health. This will necessitate the concerted efforts of professional groups and communities to learn new ways of working together and to pool their strengths and diversity for common aims. Much progress has been made to set the policy agenda and to learn about the skills required for the new ways of working. The goal now is to harness the energies and learning, and to develop new programmes of education and training to equip the workforce with the necessary skills to deliver health improvement.

References

CAIPE (1994) Defining professional and interprofessional expertise. *CAIPE, Bulletin 8* (Winter).

Chambers, J. (1997) Proposals for the first 100 days. *Health Lines*, **43**: 8.

Delaney, F. (1994) Making connections: research into intersectoral collaboration. *Health Education Journal*, **54**: 474–85.

Delaney, F. (1996) Theoretical issues in intersectoral collaboration. In Scriven, A. and Orme, J. (eds) *Health Promotion*. Basingstoke: Macmillan.

Department for Education and Employment (1997) *Excellence in Schools*. White Paper. London: DfEE.

Department for Education and Employment (1999) *National Healthy Schools Standard Guidance*. London: DfEE.

Department for the Environment, Transport and the Regions (1998) *Modernising Local Government: A New Ethical Framework*. London: HMSO.

Department for the Environment, Transport and the Regions (1999) *Implementing Best Value – a Consultation Paper on Draft Guidance*. London: HMSO.

Department for the Environment, Transport and the Regions (2000a) *The Beacon Council Scheme – Prospectus* http://www.local-regions.detr.gov.uk//beacon/prospect/2.htm

Department for the Environment, Transport and the Regions (2000b) *The Beacon Council Scheme: Application Brochure.* London: DETR.

Department of Health (1992) *The Health of the Nation.* London: HMSO.

Department of Health (1993) *Working Together for Better Health.* London: HMSO.

Department of Health (1997a) *The New NHS: Modern, Dependable.* London: HMSO.

Department of Health (1997b) *Action for Health – The Ultimate Partnership Scheme.* Press Office, DoH 97/309.

Department of Health (1998a) *Modernising Social Services.* London: HMSO.

Department of Health (1998b) *Our Healthier Nation – a Contract for Health.* London: HMSO.

Department of Health (1998c) *Partnership in Action (New Opportunities for Joint Working between Health and Social Services).* London: HMSO.

Department of Health (1998d) *Chief Medical Officer's Project to Strengthen the Public Health Function in England.* London: DoH.

Department of Health (1999a) *Saving Lives: Our Healthier Nation* (White Paper) and *Reducing Health Inequalities: an Action Report.* Health Service Circular 1999/152, Local Authority Circular (99) 26. London: DoH.

Department of Health (1999b) *Saving Lives: Our Healthier Nation.* London: Stationery Office.

Douglas, T. (1995) *Survival in Groups.* Milton Keynes: Open University Press.

Funnell, R., Oldfield, K. and Speller, V. (1995) *Towards Healthier Alliances.* London: HEA.

Grossman, R. and Scala K. (1993) *Health Promotion and Organizational Development. Developing Settings for Health.* Vienna: WHO/IFF.

Haglund, B., Borendal, B., Petterson, B., Tillgren, P. and Watson, J. (2000) Investment for health in an old mining area of Sweden. *Promotion and Education,* **VII**(2): 43–50.

Handy, C. (1995) *Gods of Management: The Changing Work of Organisations.* London: Arrow.

Health Education Authority (1998) *Piloting National Occupational Standards for Professional Activity in Health Promotion and Care. Results of the Pilot Study.* London: HEA.

Her Majesty's Stationery Office (1998) *Modern Local Government. In Touch with the People.* London: HMSO.

House of Lords Session (1995–96) Report of the Select Committee on Relations between Central and Local Government, entitled *Rebuilding Trust,* HL Paper 97.

Huczynski, A. and Buchanan, D. (1991) *Organizational Behaviour: An Introductory Text* (2nd edn). London: Prentice Hall.

Improvement and Development Agency (2000) *A Councillors's Guide to Local Government 2000.* London: IDeA.

Local Government Association (2000) *Joint Response to the Public Health White Paper, Saving Lives: Our Healthier Nation.* London: LGA/UKPHA.

Markwell, S. (1994) Building healthy alliances – the principles for success. In *Communities for Better Health.* Cardiff: Health Promotion Wales.

Markwell, S. (1998) Exploration of conflict theory as it relates to healthy alliances. In Scriven, A. (ed.) *Alliances in Health Promotion: Theory and Practice.* Basingstoke: Macmillan.

Markwell, S. (2001) Development of tools for effective working within partnership alliances, PhD to be submitted to Southampton University (in press).

National Assembly for Wales (2000) *The National Assembly for Wales*. www.better-wales.com Cardiff

National Health Service Executive (1999) *Primary Care Trusts: Establishing Better Services*. Leeds: NHSE.

National Health Service Executive (South East Region) (2000) *Strategy for Developing Public Health Capacity and Capability*. London: SERO.

Newell, T. (2000) *Forgiving Justice. A Quaker Vision for Criminal Justice*. Swarthmoor Lecture. London: Quaker Home Service.

New Opportunities Fund (1999) *Healthy Living Centres Information for Applicants*. London: NOF.

Perry, G. and Markwell, S. (2000) Promoting health in Wales – strengthening partnerships for investment for health. *Promotion and Education*, **VII**(2): 33–7.

Powell, M. (1992) *Health Alliances*. A Report to the Healthgain Standing Conference. London: King's Fund.

Royle, J., Speller, V. and Moon, A. (1999) *Exploring Interprofessional Education and Training Needs in Public Health*. Bristol: SWRO.

Sampson, E. and Marthas, M. (1981) *Group Process for Health Professionals*. Chichester: John Wiley & Sons.

Scottish Office/Department of Health (1998) *Working Together for a Healthier Scotland*. London: HMSO, and online http://www.official-documents.co.uk/document/scotsoff/hscot/

Scriven, A. (ed.) (1998) *Alliances in Health Promotion: Theory and Practice*. Basingstoke: Macmillan.

Scriven, A. and Orme, J. (eds) (1996) *Health Promotion: Professional Perspectives*. Basingstoke: Macmillan.

Social Exclusion Unit (1998) *Bringing Britain Together: A National Strategy for Neighbourhood Renewal*. London: Stationery Office.

Speller, V. (1998) Future developments of healthy alliances. In Scriven, A. (ed.) *Alliances in Health Promotion: Theory and Practice*. Basingstoke: Macmillan.

Speller, V. (1999) *Promoting Community Health: Developing the Role of Local Government*. London: HEA.

Speller, V., Markwell, S. and Scales, I. (2000) *Developing Monitoring Tools for the Pembrokeshire Alliance For Health*. Cardiff: National Assembly for Wales, Health Promotion Division (in press).

University of Reading (1994a) *MBA Making Projects Happen*. Oxford: Henley Distance Learning.

University of Reading (1994b) *MBA Organisational Development*. Oxford: Henley Distance Learning.

Watson, J., Speller, V., Markwell, S. and Platt, S. (2000) The Verona Benchmark – applying evidence to improve the quality of partnership. *Promotion and Education*, **VII**(2): 16–23.

Welsh Office (1998a) *Better Health, Better Wales. A Consultation Paper* (Cm 3922). London: Stationery Office.

Welsh Office (1998b) *Local Voices. Modernising Local Government in Wales*. Welsh Office White Paper. London: Stationery Office.

World Health Organization (1988) *Healthy Public Policy*. Geneva: WHO.

World Health Organization (1991) *Supportive Environments for Health*. Geneva: WHO.

World Health Organization (1997) *Final Report of Meeting on Policy-oriented Monitoring of Equity in Health and Health Care*. Geneva: WHO.

World Health Organization (1998a) *Review and Evaluation of Health Promotion: New Players for a New Era*. Geneva: WHO.

Ziglio, E., Hagard, S., McMahon, L., Harvey, S. and Levin, L. (2000) Principles, methodology and practices of investment for health. *Promotion and Education*, **VII**(2): 4–15.

PART II

HEALTH SERVICE

INTRODUCED AND EDITED BY JUDY ORME

Part II of this book focuses on the health service and reflects the wide range of professional activities that are a feature of health promotion within this sector. Government policy, as detailed in the modernisation agendas for the National Health Service (NHS) and local government, in particular in the White Paper *Saving Lives: Our Healthier Nation*, is focused on health improvement. Government policy clearly identifies the future role of health authorities as leading on the area health improvement. This role involves key partnership with local authorities. The role of other partners, including Primary Care Groups (PCGs) and Primary Care Trusts (PCTs), will also be crucial.

Lee Adams provides an overview of the complexities of the role of health authorities and examines the relationship between health authorities and PCGs and PCTs, discussing the opportunities for and constraints on promoting health. This chapter examines the dilemmas of partnership in the context of the government's health improvement agenda and poses some challenging questions concerning roles, responsibilities, capacity and capability.

The emergence of PCGs and PCTs is discussed in several of the chapters in Part II. In the second chapter in this section, Gill Velleman and Elizabeth Williams focus on the work of one PCG in Bristol. Their detailed insight examines the potential for implementing health promotion at a local level with particular emphasis on the PCG's role in facilitating partnership working. The two-pronged approach of working with the primary healthcare team on one-to-one interventions with patients as well as focusing on projects in the wider community is discussed. As PCTs develop, the authors argue that the aim is to retain the local focus of PCGs, with a subsequent decrease in duplication.

Cheryl Wright argues that the role of community nurses is central to the health improvement agenda and that PCGs and PCTs will be unable to achieve their objectives without the integrated contribution of these professionals. A structured approach to professional development is identified as a key consideration for the future to ensure that community nurses can work flexibly across organisational, professional and cultural boundaries.

Alyson Learmonth examines the implications of NHS reforms on specialist health promotion. The analysis of the tensions and dilemmas created for health promotion specialists who offer a unique and powerful combination of skills is particularly pertinent. The dilemmas arising from the pressure to align with primary care as against that arising from the multi-disciplinary public health agenda are clearly highlighted and discussed.

Sue Latter concludes this section by providing a detailed exploration of the potential for and barriers to health promotion in hospital nursing practice. Her chapter highlights the need for nurses to move beyond the traditional health promotion role to one that encompasses broader concepts, for example building healthy public policy, creating supportive environments and strengthening community action.

CHAPTER 3

The Role of Health Authorities in the Promotion of Health

LEE ADAMS

In this chapter, the role of health authorities (HAs) in the promotion of health will be explored, within a broad policy context that affects the public health. The remit of HAs has changed considerably over the past decade due to both Conservative and New Labour government policies, and changes are continuing with the establishment of Primary Care Trusts (PCTs). The chapter will examine the relationship of PCTs to HAs in terms of health improvement. The opportunities and constraints for HAs in promoting health will be discussed, together with the challenges they face.

The policy context

In the past decade, the NHS has undergone a major restructuring, one of many. In a sense, the NHS has been in a state of continual structural flux since its inception. However, the restructuring brought in by the Conservative government in 1990 was particularly important for HA functional change. The reforms of 1990 created what Ranude (1994) has referred to as a quasi market or managed competition. A structure of buyers and sellers was developed by separating the responsibility for the purchase of healthcare from its provision and allowing limited competition for business between providers. The Conservatives also introduced the primary care-led National Health Service (NHS) and general practitioner (GP) fundholding, creating two kinds of purchasers: HAs and GPs.

The New Labour government then produced the White Paper *The New NHS: Modern, Dependable* (DoH, 1997). The internal market was dismantled, and GP fundholding was phased out, but the government kept some of the Tory changes, notably NHS Trusts. HAs continue to plan and commission services on behalf of their populations with Primary Care Groups (PCGs). It is planned that HAs will devolve most of their commissioning function to PCTs.

Policy changes that were prioritised included: fair access to services; improved quality of provision; local responsibility putting doctors and nurses in the driving seat; partnerships between NHS organisations and also with local authorities; and greater efficiency. These changes were aimed at building confidence in the NHS as a public service that was open and accountable with public participation as a central premise.

PCGs involved teams of mainly doctors and nurses focused on natural communities. Development could occur at a number of different levels, each stage taking on more healthcare commissioning. PCGs and PCTs also have a public health function and continue as groups of practices to provide care.

Other key changes included the introduction of National Service Frameworks to improve effectiveness and efficiency, and to standardise services, and the establishment of the National Centre for Clinical Excellence to improve clinical and cost-effectiveness. A new system of clinical governance and a new Commission for Health Improvement to oversee the quality of clinical services have been developed. A new performance framework has also been introduced. Overall, HAs are poised to be leaner, with stronger powers to improve health and oversee service effectiveness.

A key duty for HAs is to lead the production of Health Improvement Programmes (HImPs). These are three-year plans that set out aims, objectives, actions and resources for health and health service improvements in the district. HImPs have to be drawn up in partnership with PCGs or PCTs, NHS Trusts and local authorities (LAs). Many of the best have also involved the voluntary and community sector. The HImP is very important as it is the framework within which all the NHS and other bodies concerned with health operate. HImPs cover health needs, healthcare requirements and the investment required to meet those needs. A later paper, *Leadership for Health* (DoH, 1999c), set out the HA role in detail.

In addition to these changes, health and social care services need to work together to provide a seamless service to the public. The NHS Act of 2000 allowed for flexibility in how funding was arranged between HAs and LAs in order to enable pooled budgets to lead commissioning and/or providing.

Local authorities are also changing and have gained new duties to improve the social, economic and environmental well-being of their communities (Local Government Act 2000). More recently, government guidance has been issued for consultation on the role and function of LAs in terms of producing Community Plans (DETR, 2000), which would encompass HImPs and other strategic plans. These changes are very important in giving LAs responsibility for public health along with HAs, and although it is not specified as such, both bodies have a role to play.

The emphasis is very much on joint planning and working. Local Strategic Partnerships are proposed to oversee Community Plans, and these will in many areas build on existing structures. Those areas which have had Healthy City partnerships or have set up Health Action Zone partnerships, and those where the HA already had a seat on a district-wide regeneration forum, will have a head start.

Promoting public health

The Conservative government produced for the first time a national health strategy, *The Health of the Nation* (DoH, 1991), which set out targets for health improvement in a number of key areas, mainly focused on disease. *The Health of the Nation* was widely criticised by the public health movement as it did not acknowledge the importance of inequalities in health and did not seek to address them. It was also largely based upon a medical model and was likely to be ineffective.

The Health of the Nation, coupled with the structural changes, had a number of effects on health promotion in and by HAs. These included the employment and management of health promotion specialists. This is discussed by Alyson Learmonth in Chapter 6. It also resulted in HA work having to focus on diseases or parts of the body instead of taking a more holistic and social approach indicated by the evidence base (Adams, 1994).

The structural changes, however, also gave those concerned with health promotion in HAs the legitimacy to set standards for providers via service agreements and to challenge the investment patterns in order to focus more on health as opposed to service improvement. Despite the hostile political climate for inequalities work and the narrow approach of the Conservative administration, it was possible to undertake evidence-based and radical work (Adams and Cunning, 2000). This was certainly the case in those areas where Healthy City or Healthy Town and Community projects were established, inspired by the WHO Health for All Agenda (WHO, 1985).

New Labour launched *Saving Lives: Our Healthier Nation*, which set out the 'third-way' approach to public health (DoH, 1999a). Inequalities were acknowledged, and a programme was set out to address them, building on a review by Sir Donald Acheson (1998). *Saving Lives: Our Healthier Nation* was welcomed for its broad vision, understanding and commitment to inequalities, its acknowledgement of the importance of a multi-disciplinary public health function and the importance of the concept of impact assessment. It also announced that Health Action Zones would be created to promote health, reduce inequalities and improve services in the most deprived areas. Twenty-six Health Action Zones have subsequently been created.

The White Paper has, however, been criticised for several reasons, including a continued limited focus on the four main action areas of cancer, heart disease, mental health and accidents. In addition, a narrow perspective is perpetuated on alleviating sickness and preventing premature death, embraced in the concept of *Saving Lives: Our Healthier Nation* (DoH, 1999a). The contribution of organisations outside the NHS was not sufficiently acknowledged. In particular, the role of LAs was felt to need more impetus. Additional criticism of the White Paper was also given for not establishing targets to reduce inequalities in health (UKPHA/LGA, 1999).

In addition, there has been a plethora of policy developed across government departments that also impacts upon health promotion practice. These include policies on sustainable development, welfare reforms, neighbourhood renewal, housing and regeneration. If they are to fulfil their functions, HAs will have to keep abreast of all such policy developments and address them with appropriate partners.

Despite the rhetoric of New Labour concerning public health improvement, their major practical focus has, however, continued to be on the NHS, waiting list reduction, financial balance, and more recently implementing the National Service Frameworks. Much energy is also being directed into supporting the establishment of PCTs. In terms of resources, it is likely that less than 1 per cent of the NHS budget is spent on health promotion, and although a key standard in the National Service Frameworks is to address inequity, this is often via what the NHS can do rather than from attention and resources being focused on attacking the root causes of ill health. The Health Action Zones, along with those areas which have Health For All initiatives (some having both), are probably best placed to keep determinants of health on the agenda for HAs. It is, however, likely that health promotion will still be marginalised because of national imperatives, a lack of appropriate skills and knowledge bases among staff and underdeveloped local infrastructures.

The role of health authorities now

Guidance in 1999 set out a radical agenda, which is a significant change of focus for HAs (DoH, 1999c). The government proposes the following:

> We want Health Authorities to embrace the modernising vision and enable all parts of the NHS to play their full part in realising it. We also want them to recognise and promote the contribution of local people, voluntary groups, and public sector partners, health and service improvements.

HAs have two key roles, first to ensure that service improvements are realised, and second to provide strategic leadership for improving health and tackling health inequalities. There is therefore much accord here with a health promotion agenda, that is, improving health, community participation, reducing inequality and intersectoral collaboration (WHO, 1981). This, together with the new duties of partnership in the NHS and in local government, means that a UK government is for the first time embracing Health for All, HAs being the leaders in this area. The guidance also outlines methods for HAs to utilise a development function and performance management. HAs can thus hold PCTs, providers and, we imagine, partners, to account for their functions as written into the HImPs.

Health authorities will no longer be spending a huge amount of time, as previously, on commissioning so could in theory spend more time on promoting health. A key approach will be ensuring that this focus is strong in the HImP and that aims lead to action. It may be that this will be challenging, as in HAs with few resources but with pressure on them to meet service imperatives. Shifting funds to health promotion would be very difficult even if this were desirable. The HImP needs to direct the service and financial framework of the NHS, the mechanism that sets out investment, if it is to be meaningful. Consideration must also be given as to how many teeth a HImP really has. The development of negotiated plans may result in an HA not being able to get an LA to act or follow its proposals through. There is a great reliance on partnership and positive relationships in the New Labour agenda. As much as this is to be applauded, partnership work is very difficult, slow and not necessarily efficient. Strategic partnerships should perhaps think collectively but then act separately (Jameson, 1999).

Health needs assessment is still a vital role for HAs. This has, however, sometimes been interpreted narrowly. Needs assessment can take many forms: utilising statistics and epidemiology is one that HAs have so far probably used as their main and sometimes only method. Participatory approaches, however, often provide more useful, accurate and rich information on which to base planning. A variety of methods can be used, but the key is the involvement at all stages of citizens and users of services (Tyrell and Harkins, 1999). It is important that marginalised communities are involved, as well as those who used to be involved before the days of participation. HAs will again need to find practical ways to make this possible. Models of good practice in the future will mean HAs working jointly with local government and the voluntary and community sectors on needs assessment to ensure that it is carried out in a planned and coherent way, and also to ensure that communities do not suffer from consultation fatigue. Community planning will certainly enable coordination. The major challenge will be to enable planning that is community owned and run to shape the agenda.

In terms of public health improvement, HAs will in their development role focus much of this on PCTs as they are on such a huge learning curve in terms of commissioning, organisational development, public health and community participation. They will, however, also need to develop the health promotion function of Trusts.

Sheffield Health was in many ways a pioneer in commissioning for health promotion, builing up good experience over several years in developing relationships with providers, Trusts, primary care and the voluntary sector. Service agreements were negotiated and performance managed carefully. In addition, programmes of development were put in place to support providers, including training, dedicated staff support time and specialist secondments. As a result, the work that some Trusts were able to do in Sheffield extended and enhanced their role in promoting health and played a role in reducing inequality in the district, as well as providing new perspectives on care and treatment. More social approaches were, for example, developed, which enhanced satisfaction with services and increased quality (Adams and Cunning, 2000).

There are difficulties with playing a development role as well as a performance management role. It can be confusing for providers, so that, despite partnerships being developed, a hard approach required by the HA to gain an improvement in compliance may not be taken seriously. However, although this is skilled work, it is highly possible to play both roles. It may be advisable that the functions are separated so that some people support and others monitor. Development work is hands on; therefore HA staff cannot be remote from delivery as they will need to work at all levels to create change.

HAs will need to ensure that services and actions aiming to improve health are effective and based upon sound evidence. This is now commonplace in many HAs but perhaps not so much in terms of their health promotion function. There is much more that could be achieved if HAs worked from the health promotion evidence base that exists. This will be particularly important in their guidance to PCTs. The Health Development Agency and Public Health Observatories will hopefully provide support for this function, but those HAs which retain a good infrastructure of health promotion specialists will be well placed to ensure effective provision and strategic work.

Although government has not set specific targets for a reduction in health inequality, HAs need to do so. For this, they will have to work as part of the community planning process, and targets should be jointly developed with LAs and with other key partners and local people; this is essential if they are to be meaningful. The government papers on neighbourhood renewal suggest that targets for neighbourhoods may be set to improve service delivery and address need. This will ensure a more effective provision and also enable effective local leadership if it is achieved with local people's involvement.

Setting local inequalities targets is, however, problematic, for several reasons, some technical and some ethical. There are also questions concerning what can be achieved at a local level when the key causes of inequality are determined nationally and, increasingly, internationally (Duggan, 2000). Again, Healthy Cities and more recently HAs have been at the cutting edge of such developments, and their learning needs to be disseminated and built upon.

Apart from strategic work with local government and the voluntary sector, HAs need to work in partnership to improve health in poor neighbourhoods and for poor and oppressed communities and population groups. The government commitment to community regeneration is very important for health improvement, although lessons from previous failed anti-poverty programmes need to be taken on board in new policies (Adams, 2001).

Area-based work will at last legitimate a health promotion focus on community development. However, although community development is a very effective way to work, it can be used in manipulative ways unless practised within a professional ethical framework. Thus, HAs need to have thought through their approaches well and ensured that good joint strategies are in place (Amos, 2000). Community development will support the development of community involvement and the extension of local democracy. The government emphasises the importance of the role of HAs in increasing local involvement in health promotion and in care services (DoH, 1999b).

Conclusion

There are many challenges for HAs in their health promotion role, not least that they need an appropriate skill and knowledge base to undertake this function. HAs will require staff with sophisticated skills in organisation and partnership development, community development and sustainable development. The ability to analyse problems, to work with all stakeholders, professionals, community groups, citizens and politicians to solve these, to plan in partnership and to bring about organisational, professional and political change is a key skill that needs to be developed.

Staff will need broad policy analysis skills and the ability to understand social, economic and environmental theory. Skills in performance management and evaluation are also vital. Strong leadership is clearly necessary from people with experience in the NHS, but also from health promotion and public health, so leaders can champion the latter as well as the former. In addition, given that many health problems require action on the root causes of ill health, skills in lobbying and influencing upwards will be required.

Government policy clearly identifies public health and health promotion as common areas needing further strengthening and recognises that health promotion programmes need to be sustained over time and be mainstreamed (DoH, 1999c).

Now is the time that HAs can really come into their own to lead strategies and to oversee the delivery of health promotion throughout their areas. To do this, considerable change is required in terms of skills to ensure that resources are available. HAs need to be bold in their health promotion function. It is an exciting time, but only time itself will tell whether HAs will be able to rise to this challenge.

References

Acheson, Sir D. (1998) *The Report of the Independent Inquiry into Inequalities in Health*. London: Stationery Office.

Adams, L. (1994) Health promotion in crisis. *Health Education Journal*, **53**: 345–60.

Adams, L. (2001) Participation – let's not mistake movement for action. *Critical Public Health* (forthcoming).

Adams, L. and Cunning, F. (2000) Promoting social and community development in Sheffield – a reflection of ten years' work. In Adams, L., Alcock, P., and Amos, M. (eds) *Promoting Health for All*. London: Sage.

Amos, M. (2000) Community development. In Adams, L., Alcock, P., and Amos, M. (eds) *Promoting Health for All*. London: Sage.

Department for the Environment, Transport and the Regions (2000) *Preparing Community Strategies. Draft Guidance to Local Authorities*. London: Stationery Office.

Department of Health (1991) *The Health of the Nation*. London: Stationery Office.

Department of Health (1997) *The New NHS: Modern, Dependable*. London: Stationery Office.

Department of Health (1999a) *Saving Lives: Our Healthier Nation*. London: Stationery Office.

Department of Health (1999b) *Patient and Public Involvement in the New NHS*. London: Stationery Office.

Department of Health (1999c) *Leadership for Health: The Health Authority Role*. London: Stationery Office.

Duggan, M. (2000) *Wakefield District HAZ, the Theoretical Base*. Wakefield: Wakefield Health Authority.

Jameson, T. (1999) *Report of a Leaders Event*. Wakefield: Wakefield Health Action Zone.

Ranude, W. (1994) *A Future for the NHS?* New York: Longman.

Tyrell, J. and Harkins, D. (1999) *Review of Participatory Needs Assessments*. Sheffield: Sheffield Health Authority.

United Kingdom Public Health Association/Local Government Association (1999) *A Response to the Acheson Report on Health Inequalities*. Birmingham: UKPHA.

World Health Organization (1981) *A Global Strategy for Health for All*. Geneva: WHO.

World Health Organization (1985) *Targets for Health for All*. Copenhagen: WHO.

CHAPTER 4

The Role of the Primary Care Group in Promoting Health

GILL VELLEMAN AND ELIZABETH WILLIAMS

In April 1999, Primary Care Groups (PCGs) were set up across England to improve the health of the population, develop primary and community services care and improve hospital services (NHS Executive, 1998a). PCGs have to set out their plans for how to achieve this role, their targets needing to reflect national priorities, local health authority priorities and the PCGs' own identification of local health issues (Primary Healthcare Development, 1999). This chapter provides a case study of the South East Bristol PCG as an example of how health promotion work has been developed within this context.

The South East Bristol PCG is one of 12 in the Avon Health Authority area and, within this, one of six covering the Bristol City Council area. All PCGs have a board of members, the board of this PCG including seven general practitioners (GPs), two nurse representatives, one social services representative, one health authority non-executive, one lay member and a chief officer. In addition, the PCG has employed an office manager and a part-time programme manager. The PCG covers a population of 67,000 and works with 12 practices, which have 40 GPs and practice staff, the local Trusts, the City Council and the voluntary sector.

Opportunities for health promotion

One of the key objectives of PCGs is to improve the health of their local population. The South East Bristol PCG is generally similar to Bristol as a whole for all the main health indicators (Avon Health Authority, 1999); there are no major illnesses, geographical areas or vulnerable groups that stand out as areas of need. For the first year of the operation of the PCG, work has focused on national, top-down priorities. These include implementing national policies at a local level, such as *Saving Lives: Our Healthier Nation* (DoH, 1999), Health Improvement Programmes (NHS Executive, 1998b; Avon Health Authority, 1999) and National Service Frameworks (DoH, 2000). The main focus is to reduce inequalities in health, heart disease, cancer, teenage pregnancies and accidents. An additional focus has been local issues that have been prioritised by the practices.

The following examples illustrate local health promotion work that was developed by the PCG between May 1999 and April 2000.

Stop smoking initiative

A major focus of national and local policies is to prevent heart disease (DoH, 2000). Smoking is the most important modifiable risk factor for coronary heart disease in the young and old (DoH, 1999). Local data demonstrate that the heart disease and smoking rates are slightly higher than the average in Avon (Avon Health Authority, 1999). The smoking cessation guidelines and their cost-effectiveness (Raw et al., 1998) contain evidence-based recommendations for the primary care team and other health professionals. This work has been extensively peer reviewed and has received wide professional endorsement. The guidelines recommend the integration of stop smoking advice into routine clinical care as one of the most important actions that a primary healthcare team can take to improve their patients' health.

A project was thus set up to:

● train health professionals to ensure that they are motivated and able to use brief interventions with smokers in an effective way;
● ensure that at least one person in each practice is trained and funded to provide further one-to-one support to smokers who want to quit;
● help practices to develop a system that delivers stop smoking interventions effectively.

This work was carried out between the PCG and the local Health Promotion Service. The first step involved an audit, which assessed what practice systems were in place to encourage giving up smoking. The audit was adapted to replicate the one developed by Yorkshire ASH/Huddersfield NHS Trust (1999). A two-page tick checklist was devised and was sent out to all local practices. The checklist detailed the provision of displays and leaflets in place, training for staff and perceived barriers. From the results, an action plan was set so all practices would have a system to deliver stop smoking interventions effectively. This contained further detail that was utilised in the training, for example addressing some of the barriers preventing health professionals from advising patients to stop smoking.

As a result the PCG and the Health Promotion Service trained 170 people. This included 75 per cent of local GPs, 71 per cent of health visitors, 38 per cent of district nurses, 71 per cent of school nurses, 80 per cent of practice nurses and 94 per cent of treatment room nurses. This training was offered in five locations and on 10 occasions. The training lasted one hour, lunch being provided. Training focused on helping staff to identify what stage of change the patients had reached, for example whether they were not ready to quit or whether they were thinking about quitting.

From the audit, one of the perceived barriers was the lack of time for staff to see patients on a one-to-one basis. The PCG had received additional funding through the modernisation fund and utilised this budget to train Support to Stop Advisers so that each practice had someone who could offer patients more support during a maximum of five one-to-one meetings. These people were then reimbursed for locum cover. The Support to Stop Advisers received more in-depth training and will continue to receive support and regular updates provided by the local Health Promotion Service and the PCG.

Each practice was provided with a smokerlyser and a nicotine replacement pack so that patients could see the range of products. Stop smoking displays were provided, which included details of the support on offer at the practice from the Support to Stop Advisers.

In addition, the PCG carried out some detailed audit work on the data produced by practice records about smoking status. The data collected could not be used to monitor trends in smoking, which is leading to work with practices in order to improve their computerised records of smoking status, as well as developing some simple computer protocols and prompts.

A comprehensive approach to stop smoking in the local practices has therefore been developed. This has included a baseline assessment of stop smoking interventions in practices an assessment of how smoking status is recorded in practices, and the development of a detailed plan to train a wide range of health professionals. Additional training has been developed so that there is a person in each practice offering further support to patients, and systems have been instigated whereby stop smoking interventions can be delivered effectively.

Reducing unwanted teenage conceptions

Reducing the number of unwanted teenage conceptions is one of the priorities set by the government. The Social Exclusion Unit's report on teenage pregnancy set two main goals (SEU, 1999):

- halving the conception rate of the under-18s and setting a firmly established downward trend in the rate for under-16s by 2010;
- achieving a reduction in the risk of long-term social exclusion of teenage parents and their children.

The PCG, focusing on the first goal, successfully bid for £3,000 from Avon Health Authority's Inequalities budget to work in this area. The PCG is expected to develop a local response to reducing teenage conceptions as part of implementing the Health Improvement Plan 2000–2003. The plan developed has taken into account the evidence of effective interventions to reduce the number of teenage conceptions (NHS Centre for Reviews and Dissemination, 1997; HEA, 1999).

An initial meeting was set up to discuss how to reduce the number of teenage conceptions. There was teaching and school nurse representation from the two local secondary schools, together with representatives from the health authority, family planning and the Health Promotion Service Avon, a local GP, a health centre receptionist, a health visitor, the PCG lay member, the head of the Bristol School Girls Mothers Unit and social services representation from two residential units. Three areas for action came out of the meeting:

1. improving personal, social and health education (PHSE) in schools;
2. improving the accessibility and acceptability of family planning services;
3. working with 'hard-to-reach' young people, such as school non-attenders and those living in residential units, as they are at greatest risk of becoming pregnant while they are teenagers.

Three groups were formed to look at these issues, and three specific action plans have been produced to take the work forward. Examples of future action include:

- Focus groups to be run in schools with school councils to determine young people's views.

- Training for teachers and school nurses on what to include in a PHSE programme and how to teach it.

- The head of the School Girls Mothers' Unit to offer a session in the school, run by a number of schoolgirl mothers, on what it is really like to have a child in your teens.

- Mapping the family planning services available to young people in the area and looking into more innovative ways of providing these services, for example having access to family planning services in the school or involving a youth worker in the provision of a family planning service.

- Offering training for GPs, practice nurses and receptionists on the most appropriate approaches and language to use with young people, particularly 'hard-to-reach' young people who want family planning services.

- Working with parents on PHSE in schools and on parenting skills, particularly with young parents, as the children of teenage parents are more likely to go on to become teenage parents.

- Offering training to staff in residential units and foster carers on sexual health issues and how they can support young people.

- Working with staff locally who are already dealing with children excluded from school or living in a residential unit on how they can help these young people to develop. Examples are careers support and self-esteem building to help them to gain more control over their lives and choose alternatives to early parenthood.

Information for patients

The PCG conducted an extensive patient satisfaction survey. Over 1,500 questionnaires were distributed to patients, resulting in 800 replies. There was a very high level of satisfaction with the services offered by the practices. However, one of the areas that respondents felt could be improved was information for patients. As a result, a group of interested practice managers and board members was established to discuss how the information available to patients in surgeries could be improved.

As a result of this project the following has been achieved:

- a named person in each practice or health centre who is responsible for patient information.

- training for these 12 individuals on how to produce eye-catching displays and notice boards.

- the purchase of extra notice boards and leaflet racks for all the practices.

- improving the notice boards by allocating different boards or parts of a board for different topics, for example practice information, PCG information, health promotion campaign literature, details of specific areas of work such as the treatment room, antenatal and post-natal information and so on. Laminated headings have been produced for all the topics.

- six health promotion displays for the practices per year on the following topics chosen by them: National No Smoking Day, healthy eating, sun awareness, stroke week, promotion of the influenza vaccine, and drink-driving. Other work of the PCG has been promoted using these displays; the no smoking display, for example, told patients about the Support to Stop person working in the practice, and the food and health display currently advertises the low-cost weight loss groups currently being piloted in the community.

- a folder listing information about 750 local self-help groups, a copy of which is placed in each waiting room for patients to look at.

One of the main advantages of working within a PCG on health promotion issues is that a local focus is possible. There are 67,000 patients registered with 12 practices; this enables relationships to be developed between the staff and the patients and response to occur to their local needs. The disadvantage of this very local model is that there is a great deal of duplication across the six PCGs in Bristol.

Promoting health from within a PCG has given greater access to primary healthcare staff, who have always been a difficult group to involve. For example, 30 out of the 40 GPs attended the smoking training described earlier. Radiating the work out from the core primary healthcare team facilitates work with other health and social services staff. Experience demonstrates that professionals such as pharmacists, dentists and road and home safety officers are keen to work on health promotion projects with the PCG. For example, as part of the accident prevention work currently being undertaken with Bristol City Council, road safety officers are providing cycling proficiency training for all year 6 pupils. Projects currently underway involve Avon Fire Brigade promoting their free smoke alarms and home fire safety checks to people over 65, as well as work with home safety officers and trading standards personnel on free electric blanket testing. Local pharmacists, dentists, post offices, community centres and sport centres have all been willing to promote these schemes.

A two-pronged approach to health promotion work involves working with the primary healthcare team on one-to-one interventions with patients, as well as setting up complementary projects in the community. Primary healthcare staff are, for example, trained to work on a one-to-one basis with people who are very overweight. At the same time, pilot work involves low-cost, self-help groups in the community to help people to lose weight. The primary healthcare staff are helping to recruit people to the self-help groups.

This multi-agency work is encouraged by the structure of the PCG board, which has representation from the health authority, the local NHS Trust, social services, general practices and the local community. Another example of this partnership working is the Falls Prevention in Older People project. A group was set up, with representation from social services, community and acute staff from the local NHS Trust, home safety, public health, health promotion and the practices. The group produced a successful bid for funding from South West Region. The project is in its infancy, but it hopes to train a wide variety of health and social services staff who work with older people in how to use a falls assessment tool to identify those at risk of falling. It will also establish agreed pathways and referral criteria for older people to receive help in preventing a fall.

The local practices in the PCG inevitably have competing and extensive demands on their time. It is essential that PCGs support surgeries so that they can implement good practice. The methods of support used are numerous. Perceived barriers to implementing health promotion programmes, which are often time and budget, are removed wherever possible. Additional funding has been used to pay the locum cost of staff time. Training is provided at a number of locations at different times, lunch being provided. It is important that PGEA approval is organised. The effective distribution of training information occurs through the practice managers, who are known personally by the PCG office. It is useful to be able to have a named person as a contact for information distribution. The simple checklist type assessment used in the smoking project did not take practices more than half an hour to complete.

The importance of the enthusiasm of the chief officer and programme manager of the PCG for evidence-based health promotion should not be overlooked. Being able to demonstrate that there is an evidence base underlying the work is very important, particularly where local health professionals feel a little jaded and unmotivated, for example in helping patients to stop smoking and lose weight. The PCG works together with health promotion specialists in the local health promotion service to plan and support health promotion work.

The PCG is ideally placed and structured to encourage partnership working, facilitating representation from many sectors to work together at a local level. The PCG ensures that there is follow-up for staff after health promotion programmes via meetings, minutes and a regular newsletter. Funding and equipment, for example smokerlysers, are provided by the PCG, which ensures that the practices have the relevant displays and leaflets. Participation in health promotion programmes is made as easy as possible for practices.

Staff in the PCG follow a very good planning process, which includes gathering the background evidence base and writing a project plan setting out the aims, objectives, timescale and evaluation. This plan is then rigorously monitored. Primary care staff are invited to be part of the planning and monitoring process, and project groups meet to review progress and decide what further steps are needed.

In summary, the PCG is able to achieve great success implementing health promotion at a local level as a result of the local contacts: the response is quick and there is an understanding of the pressure that the practices face. The PCG's role is to support people to implement the programmes with enthusiasm, but it is also an organisation that is ideally placed to implement local, successful health promotion programmes.

The six PCGs in Bristol will be consulting about becoming two Primary Care Trusts in April 2002. The aim is to maintain a local focus, as well as to reduce the duplication. The Primary Care Trust will employ a wide range of community-based staff, which should offer more opportunities for coordinated, successful health promotion programmes. The next two years will be spent setting up the structures and developing the networks to enable this to happen.

References

Avon Health Authority (1999) *Health Improvement Programme 1999/2002.* Bristol: Avon Health Authority.

Department of Health (1999) *Saving Lives: Our Healthier Nation.* London: Stationery Office.

Department of Health (2000) *National Service Framework for Coronary Heart Disease*. London: Stationery Office.

Health Education Authority (1999) *Promoting the Health of Teenage and Lone Mothers: Setting the Research Agenda*. London: HEA.

National Health Service Centre for Reviews and Dissemination (1997) *Parenting and Reducing the Adverse Effects of Unintended Teenage Pregnancies*. Effective Healthcare Bulletin, February. York: University of York.

National Health Service Executive (1998a) *Establishing PCGs*. HSC 1998/065. London: DoH.

National Health Service Executive (1998b) *Health Improvement Programmes: Planning for Better Health and Better Health Care*. HSC 1998/167. London: DoH.

Primary Healthcare Development (1999) *Simple Guide to PCG Functions*. London: Primary Healthcare Development.

Raw, M., McNeill, A. and West, R. (1998) Smoking cessation guidelines and their cost effectiveness. *Journal of the British Thoracic Society*, **53**: 5.

Social Exclusion Unit (1999) *Teenage Pregnancy*. Report CM4342. London: Stationery Office.

Yorkshire ASH/Huddersfield NHS Trust (1999) *Smoking Cessation in Practice. A Manual for Implementing the National Smoking Cessation Guidelines*. Huddersfield: Huddersfield NHS Trust.

CHAPTER 5

Community Nursing: Crossing Boundaries to Promote Health

CHERYL WRIGHT

In the White Paper *The New NHS: Modern, Dependable* (DoH, 1997) and the new public health initiative *Saving Lives: Our Healthier Nation* (DoH, 1999a), the government sets out an action plan to improve health and tackle inequalities. In order to achieve the aims detailed in these documents, new ways of working, new partnerships and interagency and multiprofessional working will be required in order to enable community nurses to deliver effective healthcare that promotes health and addresses the challenges of inequalities in health. The most radical and fundamental change is the establishment of Primary Care Groups (PCGs), and ultimately Primary Care Trusts (PCTs) as the central agents for commissioning and providing health services for local communities.

Making a Difference (DoH, 1999b) highlights the fact that community nurses are integral to improving the health of local populations, and it is evident that PCGs and PCTs will be unable to achieve their objectives without their contribution. There is an increasing acknowledgement that the context of care is changing and that nurses, midwives and health visitors face new challenges. They are often, however, constrained by structures that limit development and innovation. These include recruitment and retention problems, an ageing workforce, a rigid and constraining grading system and the need for current education and training to be updated in order to equip nurses with the full range of clinical skills needed at the point of qualification (UKCC/Commission for Nursing and Midwifery Education, 1999). Nurses of all disciplines, whether working in a community, a hospital or a primary care setting, are viewed as being crucially important to the health of local communities.

Understanding and responding to local health needs and working with local communities will become an increasingly significant aspect of professional practice. Our new vision is of professions that better reflect the communities they serve, able to provide culturally sensitive and responsive services, care and support (DoH, 1999b). The government wants to introduce new roles and develop and extend the existing roles of nurses, midwives and health visitors to make better use of their knowledge and skills; this includes more nurse-led primary care services to improve accessibility and responsiveness.

These views are supported by the report *First Assessment*, a national review of district nursing services carried out by the Audit Commission (1999). This review identified growing public demand and rising expectation, combined with changing technology and the demand for increasingly complex packages of health and social care, as well as major shifts in the policy environment that challenge district nursing services to define a clearer role. *First Assessment* also considers the opportunities that PCGs (and Local Health Groups in Wales) provide for influencing the shape of future community nursing services.

Policies and initiatives such as *Supporting Families* (Home Office, 1998), Health Improvement Programmes (HImPs), Health Action Zones (HAZs) and Healthy Living Centres (HLCs) are also being implemented to deal with a number of issues. These include chronic disease, accidents, unemployment, poor housing, pollution and family breakdown, all of which impact on health and well-being (DoH, 1999a). Such initiatives provide unprecedented opportunities for nurses and other professionals working within community settings, who do not necessarily have a tradition of working together, to improve the health of local populations by pooling their skills in innovative ways in order to promote health.

The principle underpinning this chapter is that of partnership in addition to realising the full potential of integrated teamworking by crossing organisational, professional and cultural boundaries in order to promote health through addressing the identified health needs of patients, clients and communities within the context of current government reforms.

The 10-year agenda of change

The Primary Care Act 1996 (DoH, 1996) set the agenda for improvement and development in primary care services, and the 1997 White Paper *The New NHS: Modern, Dependable* reinforced the notion of a modernised, evidence-based and primary care-led health service.

The government is developing a clear strategy for the future, based on a value driven set of initiatives. These values include:

- *partnership*: working together across the NHS to ensure the best possible care;
- *performance*: taking action to review and deliver higher standards in the NHS;
- *professions and the wider NHS workforce*: getting the right people to deliver the right services for patients and breaking down traditional barriers between healthcare professionals;

- *patient care*: speed of access and empowerment, delivering fast and convenient care for patients, listening to patients' needs and letting them know their rights;
- *prevention*: promoting healthy living across all sections of society and tackling variations in care.

In order to address these challenges, six Modernisation Action Teams have been established, led by a government minister, in order to improve performance and standards across the whole of the NHS (DoH, 2000). These values are in accordance with work carried out by Lazenbatt (1999), which explores the characteristics of successful interventions aimed at targeting health and social need. A key finding from this study is that health and social well-being is promoted through partnerships that involve collaborative working relationships and meaningful interactions between health and social care providers and the community.

A key theme running through the new government health strategy is the emphasis on integrated care and partnership working, and at the core of *Saving Lives: Our Healthier Nation* (DoH, 1999a) is the idea of a 'national contract for better health'. This recognises that health inequalities can best be tackled when individuals, families, local agencies, communities and the government work in partnership. As health needs do not recognise organisational or professional boundaries, the formation of partnerships between professionals working within and across primary, secondary and social care boundaries is essential.

Forces for change

The main drivers of change arising from the new National Health Service (NHS) agenda that impact upon community nursing on a national basis therefore include:

1. an emphasis on interagency working;
2. the increasing public health agenda focus on health promotion at a community-wide level;
3. a focus on quality, clinical effectiveness and outcomes;
4. workforce planning and training issues;
5. increased pressure on resources and changes in service demand caused by demographic, social and epidemiological factors;
6. a focus on primary care, with particular responsibility for assessing health needs (Audit Commission, 1999; UKCC/Commission for Nursing and Midwifery Education, 1999; CPHVA, 2000b).

Needs assessment

The importance of accurate assessment to identify health needs has been well documented (Peckham and Spanton, 1994; Summers and McKeowen, 1996; Timpka et al., 1996). Needs assessment is defined as:

> A systematic collection of information and data which enables the health professional to identify, analyse and prioritise the health needs and potential health needs of a given population in order to design and implement appropriate programmes of care. (Naish, 1992: 3)

This process may illustrate within a locality the extent of the poverty, deprivation, access to services, gender, age, occupation and social class of its population. Needs assessment or baseline information 'benchmark' measures are a useful yardstick against which achievement can be measured.

The World Health Organization (WHO) Alma Ata declaration of 1978 states that primary healthcare should be participative and empowering to the people and communities it serves, offering them respect and involving them in decision making. It should aim to provide local services that are community based and meet community needs. This public health approach involves working in partnership with communities to define their needs and shape services to meet those needs by cutting across disciplinary, professional and organisational boundaries (NHS Executive, 1998).

PCGs and PCTs have important new responsibilities for public health. The equitable provision of healthcare must therefore begin with a systematic assessment of the needs of the target groups and the setting of priorities in order to provide resources in the most efficient way to meet their respective needs. The available resources are not, however, always allocated equitably to assist different social groups who may be facing limited access and barriers to healthcare, perhaps of a geographical, cultural, religious or financial nature. These may include traditionally marginalised groups of people who may require health and social care but who are often difficult to identify in a population, such as travellers, the homeless community, refugees and substance abusers (Lazenbatt, 1999). It is therefore increasingly seen as essential to assess health needs in order to plan and commission effective interventions, thereby enabling teams to identify a common purpose to maximise the impact of their work (Goodwin, 1992; Twinn and Cowley, 1992; DoH, 1995; Harris, 1997).

The development of joint goals is one of the key indicators of teamwork, and developing a piece of collaborative work has been shown to increase professionals' knowledge of, and respect for, their colleagues' skills (Pritchard, 1995).

Integrated nursing teams

The need for 'joined-up' working has been highlighted in many documents and reports (Audit Commission, 1997; DoH, 1998a). As mentioned in *Modernising Health and Social Services* (DoH, 1998a), the focus must be on outcomes and how the needs of the service user are to be met. National Service Frameworks provide evidence-based care pathways that will endorse integrated working and reduce geographical variation (Hanford et al., 1999).

The Royal College of Nursing has promoted integrated nursing teams as a more effective way of meeting population needs than the traditional provision of community services. The Health Visitors Association defined an integrated nursing team as:

> A team of community based nurses from different disciplines, working together within a primary care setting pooling their skills, knowledge and ability in order to provide the most effective care for their patients within a practice and the community it covers. (Forester and Kline, 1997: 229))

Approaching problems as a team is more likely to produce creativity and a variety of potential solutions, affording the ability to integrate community care, primary care and public health (Knott, 1999).

Forester and Kline (1997) note the practical benefits, particularly to client care, that can ensue when integrated nursing teams are considered to be working well. These include a clear understanding of the different roles of team members, for example their specialist contribution, a better quality of care for the clients, including less duplication, shared protocols, an agreement on health promotion messages, the development of common audit and evaluation and effectiveness tools, allowing for a greater recognition of the qualitative aspects of care.

There has been some concern that this approach would lead to a generic community nurse and that community nurses' specialist areas of expertise would thus diminish (Pearson, 1996). Specific measures are therefore recommended to help nurses better to understand each other's philosophies, values, roles and responsibilities, as well as to promote these differences and areas of commonality to commissioners in order to develop skills in health promotion, primary prevention, community development and local public health work. Any debate in which flexibility between disciplines can be increased and restrictive professional boundaries that inhibit the promotion of health can be broken down should be welcomed. The Heathrow Debate (DoH, 1994) considered that there was in future likely to be a substitution of tasks between nurses and other professionals, and called upon nurses to be prepared to develop and change.

Witz (1994) argued that a new holistic philosophy of nursing was emerging rather than the traditional routine task-orientated approach, a philosophy supported by the Project 2000 (UKCC, 1987) initiative and enhanced by the UKCC's (1992) change in its Code of Practice. Witz (1994) argued that the future degree of autonomy to be enjoyed by nurses would depend ultimately on the ability of nurses to link this new philosophy to the new politics of health in the UK.

Royle et al. (1999) support the view that the political and clinical demands on the nursing research agenda mean that the forging of strong partnerships is crucial and that the link between the NHS and higher education remains pivotal.

New challenges and opportunities for nurses

One of the most striking features of the present government reforms is the way in which, within their policies, they have begun to capitalise on the wide skill base of nursing staff. It is therefore apparent that nurses are faced with a greater range of opportunities than ever before to expand their role, consolidate their skills and increase their influence.

A significant amount of work formerly undertaken in the acute sector is now being carried out by community-based primary care staff; hospital-at-home schemes, early discharge programmes, day surgery nurse-led minor injuries clinics, the newly established walk-in centres or triage schemes are just a few examples. These initiatives are enhanced by the increasing involvement of nurses in commissioning, nurse prescribing, clinical governance and often acting as the first point of contact with the NHS through schemes such as NHS Direct.

In the document *Shaping Tomorrow* (General Practitioner's Committee, 2000), it is emphasised that the local knowledge of community nurses should not be wasted and that better coordination and a wider use of these skills could be achieved if they had a role beyond the surgery boundary. However, the fact that community nursing is currently facing a significant recruitment and retention crisis will have a significant impact on the implementation of current government health reforms.

If nursing is to play a pivotal role in the management and provision of high-quality, cost-effective healthcare in the future, the health service must be able to recruit a sufficient number of nurses to meet government health policy objectives, but employers are experiencing increasing difficulties in recruiting qualified staff. The number of nursing students entering training has dropped by a third since the late 1980s, with a decline in the number of newly qualified nurses and midwives registering with the UKCC between 1993–94 and 1997–98. Another factor set to reduce this diminishing pool even further is the disproportionately large number of nurses who will retire within the next five years, one in 10 of those registered being 55 years old or over (Audit Commission, 1999; UKCC/Commission for Nursing and Midwifery Education, 1999; General Practitioner's Committee, 2000).

The current trend of a national shortage of nursing personnel may be caused by the perception of nursing as an unattractive profession and of the low value of caring/women's work. The Director General of WHO noted in 1992:

> Until society values caring work and women's work more highly, and rewards them accordingly, measures taken to attract new recruits will not succeed; well educated, motivated women will continue to seek careers in occupations that have a higher social standing and higher remuneration. The social consequences of this for the health and well-being of populations will be disastrous. (Warner et al., 1998: 24)

Around 27 per cent of health visitors are also due to retire over the next five years, the same being true in school nursing and district nursing (DoH, 1999b). In recent years, some health authorities have questioned the value of health visitors. The government's public health agenda has, however, provided health visitors with the potential to become one of the central players in delivering the new vision for health through a family-centred public health role.

The *Supporting Families* strategy (Home Office, 1998) has important implications for community nurses, signalling in particular an expanded role for health visitors. During the past 10 years, the focus of health visiting practice has been determined by contracts commissioned by general practitioner fundholders and health authorities. This has constrained the range of activities and skills offered by health visitors, especially this public health role.

The particular skills of health visitors span health promotion and health needs assessment with individuals, families, communities and populations. PCGs and other partner organisations, including the voluntary sector, will therefore be increasingly looking to health visitors to lead and facilitate preventative strategies and to articulate their unique contribution to the coordination of health promotion and health needs assessment.

There are, however, significant challenges that may hamper the ability of the profession to deliver the outcomes required by the new agendas. These include tackling workforce pressures and maintaining and developing appropriate training and education structures (CPHVA, 2000a). These challenges are further emphasised in *Making a Difference* (DoH, 1999b).

A recent study commissioned by the UKCC and the Commission for Nursing and Midwifery Education (1999), in order to propose a way forward for pre-registration education that enabled fitness for practice based on healthcare need, identified a number of trends that look set to continue. This includes an ageing population, changing professional roles and changing workforce expectations. Another key issue identified was the need to move towards interprofessional learning and working.

Interprofessional education and training

Interprofessional education and training is seen as a way of establishing relationships with and promoting collaboration between different disciplinary
groups (Royle et al., 1999). The importance of learning shared with other
community nurses, reflecting a wider health and social care interface, is also
emphasised by Oldman (1999). This is further supported by the strategy for
nurses, midwives and health visitors requiring educational programmes to
prepare them to contribute fully to a modern NHS (DoH, 1999b). This
document supports the view that the political and clinical demands on the
nursing research agenda mean the forging of strong partnerships and links
between the clinical and academic is crucial.

To deliver patient care and meet the health needs of the new millennium,
we have to ensure that health professionals working within the wider health
and social care community have the right education, training, skills and
opportunities further to develop their existing skills. It is also crucial to create
a profile of the knowledge, skills and competencies of all healthcare professionals working within a locality and link this to the local HImP.

Health Improvement Programmes

HImPs are three-year plans that provide the key vehicle for the government
to achieve its principal objectives of tackling health inequalities and securing
an improvement in the four national priority areas (heart disease and stroke,
accidents, cancer and mental health), in addition to responding to local priorities. A recent review of national health improvement programmes by Abbott
and Gillam (2000), however, found a wealth of priorities reflecting national
policy, but measurable targets were very thin on the ground. The study
sought evidence of a commitment to national and local priorities for health
improvement, public consultation and partnership working, a strategy driven
by health needs and effective implementation of the strategy.

The approach to HImPs is underpinned by partnership working and new
statutory duties upon health organisations and local authorities to work
together to improve the health and well-being of communities through a
national contract for health improvement.

Health Action Zones

HAZs are 26 area-based partnerships established to pioneer creative
approaches to tackling health inequalities and modernising services via innovative health-promoting initiatives.

While all HAZs share problems of deprivation and poor health, they vary
considerably in terms of their size, organisational complexity and population

profile. The difference between HAZs has important implications for assessing the effectiveness, efficiency and sustainability of health-promoting services such as smoking cessation.

Adams et al. (2000), in their presentation of preliminary findings relating to the introduction of smoking cessation services in HAZs, stipulate that it will be essential to balance this capacity for innovation with the delivery of effective and sustainable services in the future. They warn that, although the current government appears to be committed to modernisation at a rapid pace, real and sustained results will not be achieved unless sensible foundations are laid at an early stage of development. The potential barriers identified to the design and implementation of effective service delivery systems include: a lack of clarity on the organisation of services; establishing monitoring systems; involving PCGs and other agencies in planning and delivering services; and recruiting and retaining qualified staff (Adams et al., 2000). Community development is specifically identified as the underlying methodology in HAZ work (CPHVA, 2000b).

Healthy Living Centres

HLCs provide a real opportunity to improve health and reduce inequalities in health through local community action. The overall objective of the New Opportunities Fund is, by September 2002, to commit funds to projects that between them should establish or develop HLCs with a total catchment area covering around 20 per cent of the population of the UK. Funding for individual projects should in general last for no more than five years.

There will be no standard blueprint for projects. The initiative is designed to encourage innovative proposals that will respond to the varying needs of different communities and groups. The programme will in the first instance target the most deprived areas. HLCs will be expected to show how they complement HImPs and contribute to achieving local health priorities (NHS Executive, 1999). The initiative is complementary to *Saving Lives: Our Healthier Nation* (DoH, 1999a) and will focus on health in its broadest sense, providing the opportunity to improve quality of life and enable people to achieve their full potential.

HLCs can include a range of models and are most importantly about initiatives, partnerships and networks rather than bricks and mortar. HLCs provide scope to assist PCGs in achieving their objectives. The contact that the range of primary care practitioners, including community nurses, has with their local communities should enable them to make an important contribution to the development of local proposals based on real needs.

HLCs are expected to be able to demonstrate new ways of working across current boundaries and innovative approaches to providing the opportunity for people to improve their health and well-being. They are to be the focus for interagency action for community health improvement at a local level.

Clinical effectiveness

The influence of NHS policy-making processes, raised public expectations of healthcare provision and the changing demography of the population all exert pressure on and offer a challenge to community nursing professionals working within today's primary care-led NHS. Community nurses need to have supportive infrastructures that will allow them to respond to identified health needs and inform the commissioning agenda of PCTs, deal with increasing demands and find innovative ways of providing clinically effective services.

As clinical governance is being implemented (DoH, 1998b), with clinically effective working practices as a core theme, the practical aspects of interprofessional working and learning become even more important. We need to understand the implications of interprofessional working and learning, and recognise how best to develop its potential. Above all, services should be responsive to the needs of the patient and build upon the skills of practitioners.

Recurring themes permeating the current health policy agenda are the need to:

- increase the attention given to health promotion and disease prevention services;
- maximise the attention given to clinical effectiveness in service planning and delivery in order to continue to improve the quality of care;
- ensure that services respond to and are focused on need.

It is crucial that the change process is supported and safe practice is ensured through mechanisms such as clinical supervision. Clinical supervision is an important professional relationship for increasing clinical effectiveness and for supporting and enabling the new initiative of clinical governance in the NHS (RCN, 1999). Clinical effectiveness has been defined by the NHS Executive (1996: 7) as:

> The extent to which specific clinical interventions when deployed in the field for a particular patient or population, do what they are intended to do, that is, maintain and improve health and secure the greatest possible health gain.

Clinical supervision should properly be seen as taking its place in the wider framework of activities that are designed to promote health and monitor the delivery of high-quality health-promoting activities.

Community development

Community development emphasises the importance of public participation in health-promoting activities by defining health needs, crossing professional boundaries and bringing community practitioners and organisations together (Twinn and Cowley, 1992). In 1995, the Standing Nursing and Midwifery Advisory Committee published a report on the contribution of health visitors, nurses and midwives to public health. *Making it Happen* (DoH, 1995) spelt out the many key areas in which, based on the health-promoting principles of health visiting, all nursing disciplines can make a contribution to public health initiatives (CETHV, 1977). These included:

- a knowledge of local communities;
- working with whole communities, using established networks across the voluntary and statutory sectors;
- identifying health needs, assessing outcome and evaluating effectiveness and acceptability.

The close link between the aims and practices of community development and public health suggests that community nurses are well placed to be undertaking this kind of work.

Primary Care Groups: Delivering the Agenda (DOH, 1998c) sets out the PCG's health improvement role. From April 1999, all PCGs are expected to improve the health of, and address health inequalities in, their community. This will involve harnessing the skills of community nursing staff with particular regard to assessing health needs in order to contribute to the development of the local HImPs and HAZ plans.

Conclusion

Community nurses are continuing to work in new ways in order to meet increasingly diverse healthcare needs, and are assuming a stronger health promotional role. They are also forming stronger commissioning partnerships with other members of PCGs and PCTs. Elsewhere in the community, nurses are working in a variety of settings in order to engage in a range of health-promoting activities. This facilitates the growing emphasis on both working and learning together. Professionals such as primary care liaison nurses, health and social care team coordinators and nurse practitioners are also now working across the spectrum of clinical practice between the community and hospital sector.

The government has recognised the importance of shifting the spotlight onto the community in order to achieve its health policy objectives. Community nursing, with its focus on health promotion and community profiling, is an excellent basis on which to develop the essential combination of skills and knowledge required for the future commissioning and provision of health services. The supply of qualified nurses has not, however, kept pace with demand. Based on the available evidence on the value of nursing and the impact of innovations in nursing practice, the health services need more nurses if the health needs of tomorrow's population are to be met.

Teamwork within community nursing must therefore be viewed in a wider perspective than that of solely the nursing team if the effective promotion of health is to occur. The full range of services, agencies and healthcare professions needs to be engaged, and all available skills harnessed, in order to address health needs effectively. This means that a structured approach to professional development is needed in order to broaden and identify transferable skills within existing roles in addition to enabling staff to meet the challenges of a primary care-led NHS and to work more flexibly in future.

Community nursing staff are only too well aware of the increasing expectations placed upon them. It is therefore crucial to re-examine the current organisation of service delivery, to identify strengths and gaps, and to aim to build on the strengths.

References

Abbott, S. and Gillam, S. (2000) Trusting to luck. *Health Service Journal*, 110(5705): 24–5.

Adams, C., Bauld, L. and Judge, K. (2000) Baccy to front. *Health Service Journal*, 110(5713): 28–31.

Audit Commission (1999) *First Assessment: A Review of District Nursing Services in England and Wales.* London: Audit Commission for Local Authorities and the National Health Service in England and Wales.

Community Practitioners and Health Visitor's Association (2000a) *Leading the Future: A Report on a Simulation-based Enquiry into the Future of Health Visiting.* London: Office for Public Management.

Community Practitioner's and Health Visitor's Association (2000b) *Joined Up Working: Community Development in Primary Health Care.* London: CPHVA.

Council for the Education and Training of Health Visitors (1977) *The Principles of Health Visiting.* London: CETHV.

Department of Health (1994) *The Challenges for Nursing and Midwifery in the 21st Century (The Heathrow Debate).* London: DoH.

Department of Health, Standing Nursing and Midwifery Advisory Committee (1995) *Making it Happen.* London: HMSO.

Department of Health (1996) *Primary Care Act.* London: HMSO.

Department of Health (1997) *The New NHS: Modern, Dependable.* London: HMSO.

Department of Health (1998a) *Modernising Health and Social Services: National Priorities Guidance.* London: HMSO.

Department of Health (1998b) *A First Class Service: Quality in the New NHS.* London: DoH.

Department of Health (1998c) *Primary Care Groups: Delivering the Agenda.* HSC 1998/228. Edinburgh: Churchill Livingstone.

Department of Health (1999a) *Saving Lives: Our Healthier Nation.* London: HMSO.

Department of Health (1999b) *Making a Difference. Strengthening the Nursing, Midwifery and Health Visiting Contribution to Health and Healthcare.* London: HMSO.

Department of Health (2000) *The National Plan for the New NHS: Challenges Facing the National Health Service.* http://www.nhs.uk/nationalplan/challenges.htm (accessed 6 June).

Forester, S. and Kline, R. (1997) Integrated nursing teams. *Health Visitor,* **70**(6): 229–31.

General Practitioner's Committee (2000) *Shaping Tomorrow: Issues Facing General Practice in the New Millennium.* London: BMA.

Goodwin, S. (1992) Community nursing and the new public health. *Health Visitor,* **64**(9): 294–6.

Hanford, L., Easterbrook, L. and Stevenson, J. (1999) *Rehabilitation for Older People: The Emerging Policy Agenda.* London: King's Fund.

Harris, A. (ed.) (1997) *Needs to Know: A Guide to Needs Assessment for Primary Health Care.* Edinburgh: Churchill Livingstone.

Home Office (1998) *Supporting Families: A Consultation Document.* London: HMSO.

Knott, M. (1999) Integrated nursing teams: developments in general practice. *Community Practitioner,* **72**(2): 23–4.

Lazenbatt, A. (1999) *Targeting Health and Social Need: Manual for Evaluation in Practice* (Vol. 2). Belfast: Queen's University of Belfast.

Naish, J. (1992) *Profiling School Health.* London: HVA.

National Health Service Executive (1996) *Promoting Clinical Effectiveness – a Framework for Action in and Through the NHS.* Leeds: DoH.

National Health Service Executive (1998) *In the Public Interest: Developing a Strategy for Public Participation in the NHS.* Leeds: NHSE/Institute of Health Service Management/NHS Confederation.

National Health Service Executive (1999) *Healthy Living Centres.* Health Service Circular HSC 1999/008. Leeds: DoH.

Oldman, C. (1999) An evaluation of health visitor education in England. *Community Practitioner,* **12**(12): 392–5.

Pearson, P. (1996) Towards a primary care-led NHS. *Health Visitor,* **69**(9): 376–8.

Peckham, S. and Spanton, J. (1994) Community development approaches to health needs assessment. *Health Visitor,* **67**(4): 124–5.

Pritchard, P. (1995) Learning to work effectively in teams. In Owens, P., Carrier, J. and Herder, J. (eds) *Interprofessional Working in Community and Primary Health Care.* London: Macmillan.

Royal College of Nursing (1999) *Realising Clinical Effectiveness and Clinical Governance through Clinical Supervision. The Practitioner's Companion, Part 2.* Oxford: Radcliffe Medical Press.

Royle, J., Speller, V. and Moon, A. (1999) *Exploring Interprofessional Education and Training Needs in Public Health.* Bristol: NHS Executive South West Region.

Summers, A. and McKeowen, K. (1996) Health needs assessment in primary care: a role for health visitors. *Health Visitor,* **69**(8): 323–4.

Timpka, T., Svensson, B. and Molin, B. (1996) Development of community nursing: analysis of the central services and practice dilemmas. *International Journal of Nursing Studies,* **33**(7): 297–308.

Twinn, S. and Cowley, S. (1992) *The Principles of Health Visiting: A Re-examination.* London: HVA.

United Kingdom Central Council for Nursing, Midwifery and Health Visiting (1987) *Project 2000: The Final Proposals.* London: UKCC.

United Kingdom Central Council for Nursing, Midwifery and Health Visiting (1992) *The Scope of Professional Practice.* London: UKCC.

United Kingdom Central Council for Nursing, Midwifery and Health Visiting/ Commission for Nursing and Midwifery Education (1999) *Fitness for Practice*. London: UKCC.

Warner, M., Longley, M., Gould, E. and Picek, A. (1998) *Healthcare Futures 2010*. University of Glamorgan: Welsh Institute for Health and Social Care. (Commissioned by the UKCC Education Commission.)

Witz, A. (1994) The challenge of nursing. In Gabe, J., Kellner, D. and Williams, G. (eds) *Challenging Medicine*. London: Routledge.

World Health Organization (1978) The Alma Ata Declaration. *World Health Organization Chronicle*: **32**: 28–9.

World Health Organization (1992) More than Ever we Need Nurses (editorial). *World Health*, Sept–Oct.

CHAPTER 6

The Role of Specialist Health Promotion Services

ALYSON LEARMONTH

When the previous edition of this book was published in 1996, Linda Ewles finished her chapter on 'The impact of the NHS reforms on specialist health promotion in the NHS' as follows:

> It is arguable that their future depends on the key ingredients of increased profes-
> sionalism, evidence of effectiveness, investment in larger departments and a
> prolonged period of organisational stability. (Ewles, 1996: 73)

Four years later, those themes are still with us, although the context has changed dramatically. This chapter looks at the implications of these changes for specialists in health promotion. First, it may be useful to define the role and functions of specialist health promotion services. The 'professional perspective' theme of this book is represented for specialists in health promotion in the UK through the Society for Health Education and Promotion Specialists (SHEPS), which was founded in 1982.

Role and function of specialist health promotion services in the UK

The World Health Organization currently offers the following definition of health promotion:

> Health promotion is the process of enabling people to increase control over, and
> to improve their health.
>   Health promotion represents a comprehensive social and political process, it not
> only embraces actions directed at strengthening the skills and capabilities of indi-
> viduals, but also action directed towards changing social, environmental and
> economic conditions so as to alleviate their impact on public and individual health.
> (WHO, 1998: 1)

The glossary goes on to reaffirm the priority areas defined in the Ottawa Charter (WHO, 1986):

- building public policies that support health;
- creating supportive environments;
- strengthening community action;
- developing personal skills;
- reorienting health services.

It then adds the Jakarta Declaration priorities for health promotion in the 21st century:

- Promote social responsibility for health.
- Increase investment for health development.
- Expand partnerships for health promotion.
- Increase community capacity and empower the individual.
- Secure an infrastructure for health promotion.

The UK is well placed in relation to the last of these points. Health promotion specialists are an identified workforce whose specific purpose is to promote health, through the whole range of activities advocated by the World Health Organization (WHO). Health promotion specialists see themselves as:

> advisors, consultants, researchers, trainers, project leaders, coordinators, policy development officers, enablers, mediators and advocates. Through these roles they help many thousands of workers such as doctors, nurses, teachers, police officers, Local Authority representatives, company directors and community representatives to carry out health promotion work within their own setting. Health Promotion Specialists are the key catalysts and facilitators for the vast majority of health promotion work carried out within the UK, for which our country has a deservedly high reputation. (SHEPS, 1999: 4)

The key words here are 'catalysts' and 'facilitators' as these ideas are central to an understanding of the role of health promotion specialists.

In practice, however, what sorts of activity do health promotion specialists undertake? The exact service profile varies according to local circumstances, but activities are likely to fall into the following clusters:

1. Organisational development:
   - leadership
   - partnership development
   - training, education and support
   - policy and strategy development

- evidence-based practice
- market research, communication and publicity
- programme management.

2. Community development:
  - advocacy
  - needs assessment
  - community participation
  - information for health
  - evaluation.

While not exclusive to health promotion specialists, the skills shown in this list create a unique and powerful combination.

In practical terms, where are health promotion specialists located? In 1999, a survey into the organisational positioning and staffing of 153 health promotion departments in the UK was carried out, an analysis being produced based on the 108 completed questionnaires that were received (Robertson and Macdonald, 2000). The results of the survey can be compared with those from an earlier piece of work in order to track changes in the field (Milner and French, 1997).

The first striking point is the level of organisational change being experienced: since 1990, the organisational position has changed for all specialist health promotion services in Wales and Northern Ireland, for over two-thirds in England and for over half in Scotland. It is clear that the period of stability advocated by Linda Ewles in the quote at the start of this chapter has been far from the actual experience.

In 1996, there was a continuing trend to locate specialist health promotion departments in Trusts. There is evidence that this trend is now reversing, and that in England there is a shift to working more closely with Primary Care Groups (PCGs). Compared with 1996, there now seem to be fewer fixed-term contracts. Over the past two years, it would seem that about a third of health promotion departments have seen an increase in their staffing level while about a third have seen a decrease. The average funding per head of population has increased from £1.23 in 1996 to £1.38 in 1999, which is less than the rate of inflation. There is still a wide range, from £0.46 to £7.00 per person, although the funding ratio is, overall, better in Scotland.

Finally, to complete this profile of specialist health promotion services, it is worth discussing the status of the group as a profession. SHEPS members follow a Code of Professional Practice and have a Principles of Practice group, SHEPS also has criteria for acknowledging the academic courses that form the foundation of theory, which is used by health promotion specialists to inform their practice. About two-thirds of health promotion specialists hold a postgraduate qualification in either health promotion or public health (Robertson and MacDonald, 2000).

There are two deficits in the requirements for recognition as a profession. One is an accepted national scheme for postgraduate accreditation and recognition, the second a linked requirement for the registration of practising health promotion specialists. This second issue has in the past generated a vigorous debate between some members of SHEPS who saw it as a means to professional recognition, and others for whom it implied elitist exclusivity. At the time of writing, this issue is again under active consideration by SHEPS members (SHEPS, 2000).

Multi-disciplinary public health and partnership working

Saving Lives: Our Healthier Nation (DoH, 1999a) declares a strategic intention that a modern public health workforce will be made up of people from many different backgrounds. This workforce needs to be able to:

- manage strategic change;
- act as the leaders and champions of public health;
- work in partnership with other agencies and individuals;
- develop communities with a focus on health;
- be familiar with public health concepts and, where appropriate, use evidence in guiding their own work;
- apply their professional skills and knowledge in order to play a part in securing the aims set out in the White Paper (paragraph 11.9).

The White Paper also makes the statement that, within the National Health Service (NHS), the post of Specialist in Public Health will be created, equivalent in status for independent practice to medically qualified consultants in public health medicine, able to become Directors of Public Health (paragraph 11.25). This is a major step in one sense, yet at the same time it assumes a 'gold standard' provided by training in public health medicine rather than an open access, multi-route system of accreditation related equally to all five areas of the Ottawa Charter principles quoted earlier.

While English policy in relation to this specific aspect of multi-disciplinary public health has gone furthest, there are active developments in this area occurring also in Wales (1998) and Scotland (2000), and changes anticipated in Northern Ireland. This has led to a flurry of activity both through the Health Development Agency and the NHS Executive, working with the Faculty of Public Health Medicine, the Royal Society of Health and the Multidisciplinary Public Health Forum (Healthwork UK, 2000). The terms of reference for this activity were set by the interim findings of the Chief Medical Officer's review (1998), which identifies three levels of involvement in public health:

- professionals who would benefit from a better understanding of public health;
- a smaller group of hands-on public health practitioners who spend a substantial part of their working time furthering health by working with communities and groups;
- a still smaller group of public health specialists from a variety of professional backgrounds, with the ability to manage strategic change and lead public health initiatives.

Health promotion specialists are given as an example of the second group, although health promotion is recognised as a source discipline for public health specialists. This categorisation is at variance with the WHO concept of health promotion and the view of many health promotion specialists in the field in the UK.

At the same time as the wealth of activity in relation to defining competencies and routes to accreditation for a multi-disciplinary public health workforce, there is also a strong drive at a national level in terms of 'joined-up thinking'. This is reflected in various ways, one being the creation of new posts and roles. There is, for example, an Under Secretary for Public Health. The Health Development Agency, established from April 2000, has a remit that includes:

> advising on the setting of standards for public health and health promotion practice, and on the implementation of those standards by a range of organisations at national and local level. (DoH, 1999a: 129)

The Social Exclusion Unit has a specific brief to work across government departments and has now produced 18 reports with wide-ranging implications, culminating in the *National Strategy for Neighbourhood Renewal: a Framework for Consultation* (SEU, 2000). One of their more specific areas of work, which has already had a direct impact on many health promotion specialists in England, is the report on *Teenage Pregnancy* (SEU, 1999).

Nationally, the policy agenda is vast, embracing on the one hand such specific areas of concern as tobacco control (DoH, 1998a), and on the other a raft of initiatives related to education, housing, modernising local democracy and so on (Miller, 1998). At a local level, the Health Improvement Programme (HImP) provides a mechanism for coordinating and leading partnership work related to health and well-being rather than just the prevention of illness.

Opportunities in relation to multi-disciplinary public health

There is clearly a context of national and local policy-led change related to the wide arena of issues of concern in health development, with a focus on redressing social exclusion. This presents a tremendous opportunity for specialists in health promotion to play a part in bringing about the changes they have long advocated.

There is also the linked opportunity for health promotion specialists to make an important contribution to the development of the multi-disciplinary public health task force required by national policy. The WHO principles for health promotion in terms of equity and participation make health promotion specialists committed to involving the whole range of public health workers in discussing needs, identifying competencies and developing accreditation pathways.

In the meantime, some specialist health promotion services are combining with their colleagues in public health medicine to form the start of new multi-disciplinary departments of public health, which will act as core players in the new health authority role as defined in *Leadership for Health* (DoH, 1999b). At a minimum, this shift reverses the split that was widely experienced when health promotion was organisationally separated from public health during the creation of the purchaser–provider split during the early-to-mid 1990s. In the longer term, it may lead to joint services with local authorities, consolidating the partnership approach. Even where this is not happening, there is no doubt that the fiercely competitive and number-crunching aspects of the contract culture are disappearing, so that collaboration across organisational boundaries is easier than when the previous edition of this book was published.

Constraints in relation to multi-disciplinary public health

There is a risk in terms of the current focus of activity that energy is diverted into the question of equivalence between medical and non-medical public health specialists. That this debate is a real one to those involved is clear, not least because of the considerable pay differential involved, ranging from £17,000–20,000 for a health promotion specialist and £25,000–40,000 for a health promotion manager to £44,000–58,000 for a public health consultant (French, 1999). It may, however, seem navel gazing to partners in other agencies that the supposed advocates of partnership working are tangled up in questions of pay and status.

For health promotion specialists, the lack of professional recognition may be serious. In the worst case scenario, it could mean that in order to 'become' a 'public health specialist', an entire process of retraining would have to be undertaken according to the criteria of the Faculty of Public Health Medicine. This would be a waste of existing experience and expertise, as well as a failure to recognise the unique contribution that specialists in health promotion may make in their own right.

Finally, there is a concern that the partnership working being advocated is not supported by adequate indicators of process, to encourage robust developments on the ground. The steps in developing partnership working have been well documented (Funnell et al., 1995), but there has to date been little evidence that measures of commitment, resources, shared vision, participation and accountability are being taken seriously as the building blocks of effective 'joined-up working' on the ground. It may be that the new role of the Health Development Agency in setting appropriate standards for multi-disciplinary health at an organisational level may come into play in relation to this issue.

The role of primary care collectives

The second theme is the developing health promotion role of collective representation, negotiation and commissioning on the part of primary care. The terms of reference for primary care groups include (DoH, 1998b):

- promoting the health of the local population;
- working in partnership with other agencies;
- reflecting the perspective of the local community and the experience of patients;
- providing a forum for professional development, audit and peer review;
- contributing to HImPs (all from section 5.9);
- playing an active part in community development (section 5.27);
- possessing effective arrangements for public involvement (section 4.19);
- making choices about the cost-effective provision of service (section 5.30).

There are equivalent moves in relation to Local Healthcare Cooperatives in Scotland (Chief Medical Officer's Review, 2000) and Local Health Groups in Wales (Welsh Office, 1998). This range of functions clearly means that primary care collectives have a strong role to play in promoting the health of the population, from a primary care perspective, through their arrangements with secondary care providers and working in partnership with local authority and voluntary sector colleagues. A creative interface with specialist health promotion services to assist them in these three areas of work is therefore crucial.

As PCGs increasingly become Primary Care Trusts (PCTs), their autonomy from the health authority in developing these functions will increase. The currently popular organisational solution of attaching 'named' specialists to each PCG from a central health authority- or Trust-based service will become harder to sustain. At the same time, as most PCGs serve populations of around 100,000, they are unlikely without significant investment to be able to support a specialist health promotion service on a stand-alone basis. Furthermore, the case for the total devolution of specialist health promotion services to PCGs risks a loss of work at a strategic level with the health authority in relation to the roles described in the first section of this chapter.

Opportunities in relation to primary care collectives

The role of PCGs, Local Healthcare Cooperatives and Local Health Groups may release fresh energy into the development of opportunities to promote health via the primary care team. They may also influence more effectively than has been possible in the past the development of health-promoting practice as part of the role of PCTs. Looking to the future, work covering a population of 100,000 people might also provide a natural level for partnership working with local authorities, especially where the boundaries are co-terminous. This level of working may become increasingly important if the possible scenario of health authority mergers (as their purchasing role is taken over by PCTs) materialises.

Constraints in relation to the role of primary care collectives

The survey of specialist health promotion resources quoted above suggests that there has been little real growth and development over the past 3–4 years. Specialist health promotion services will not be able to function adequately if they are 'divided up' between PCGs/PCTs without any of the following:

● a specialist health promotion service manager capable of working at a strategic level;
● groups large enough to provide a good skill mix, and be able to work in a range of settings with the capacity for training and developing staff;
● the board or Trust understanding the capacity-building nature of the service;
● clear arrangements for partnership working in all sectors.

Even if these criteria are met, the picture is one in which the tension arising from the pressure to align with primary care, offset against that arising from the multi-disciplinary public health agenda, is likely to create increasingly diverse circumstances in which health promotion specialists will find themselves working.

Evidence of effectiveness and innovation

This leads into the third theme addressing the environment currently shaping specialists in health promotion services. Over the past decade, there has been increasing pressure in relation to the question of evidence-based practice as it applies to the activity of promoting health (Speller et al., 1997). Three major developments in this area seem likely to shape the future development of what is accepted as core good practice.

The first is the development of the concept of clinical governance:

> Clinical governance provides a framework within which local organisations can work to improve and assure the quality of clinical services to patients. (DoH, 1999b: 3)

While the focus is on clinical outcomes, clinical governance is about developing people, teams and systems (Chambers, 1999). As PCGs and PCTs begin to address the issues of wider accountability involved in clinical governance, they may increasingly call on the experience of health promotion specialists in bridging the gap from a purely biomedical model to collaborative working and participative methods.

The second development is the creation of National Service Frameworks, which are intended to:

> set out the vision for the future and the practical short and medium term actions required to achieve that vision. They will evolve as new evidence becomes available. (DoH, 2000: 5)

Both *Mental Health* (DoH, 1999c) and *Coronary Heart Disease* (DoH, 2000) have their first standard concerned with health promotion/prevention. Once recommendations are included in the frameworks, the arguments about whether the practice is justified and effective can be laid to one side.

Both these frameworks have been prepared in advance of the initiation of the Health Development Agency, which has as a key role:

> maintaining an up to date map of the evidence base for public health and health improvement. (DoH, 1999a: 129)

An initial start to this task has been made with the publication of the discussion document *Evidence Base 2000: Evidence into Practice* (Gillies, 1999). This proposes an approach to evidence-based practice that, where appropriate, draws on non-experimental studies, for example ethnographic studies, case studies, action research and so on. It also lays out a conceptual framework for seeking and mapping evidence based on three perspectives: evaluation and effectiveness, best practice and action research. All three aspects revolve around an axis focusing on vulnerable groups and assessing progress in relation to inequalities in health. If this approach is successfully developed, there will be for the first time a national body in England sifting and making available evidence from the variety of sources that health promotion specialists have been advocating for some time (Learmonth and Watson, 1999).

The second half of this theme though concerns innovation. This is included alongside a discussion of evidence-based practice because the pace of technological change at times means that only the broadest principles of good practice are available to help to inform what may be quite major shifts in policy direction and service development.

An example may serve to illustrate this point – the move towards reducing drastically the amount of printed and audio-visual material that has traditionally been one of the defining functions associated with most (although not all) specialist health promotion services. The rationale is clear in terms of electronic communication and the possibilities for personal advice and information opened up by NHS Direct. Yet making the change at a pace and in a way that does not yet again disadvantage those in our society with least resources is far less clear. The changes proposed are certainly not evidence based.

Opportunities in relation to evidence of effectiveness and innovation

The Health Development Agency role for the first time gives a clear national lead in England to the question of developing evidence-based practice. This will save the repetitious and under-resourced efforts of specialists in health promotion locally in trying to carry out local assessments of evidence in relation to programmes of activity. It also provides a vehicle by which studies can be commissioned to address the relatively neglected areas of research into health policy, organisational development and community-capacity building rather than the much focused-on lifestyle changes resulting from one-to-one interactions with patients.

Another opportunity may arise in the development of clinical governance. Since few choices can be made on the basis of scientific information alone, methods of decision making based on respecting and working with the values of others are likely to be in high demand. National Service Frameworks provide a chance for at least some aspects of health promotion activity to be regarded as firm requirements rather than the subject of debate.

Constraints

While the three developments discussed all create a context in which an appropriate evaluation of health promotion activity may develop, it must still be recognised that practical decision making is based on realpolitik as much as evidence. In this scenario, the Health Development Agency role is crucially political at all levels – with senior government, with the range of professional groups and organisations that form part of a multi-disciplinary public health workforce, with the fieldworkers themselves and with the public.

Conclusion

To conclude, the pace of change affecting specialist health promotion services continues to be frantic. The constraints concern mainly capacity, location and recognition. Delivering on the agenda presented requires the development of a truly multi-disciplinary public health workforce, with accreditation processes that are clear, openly accessible, self-regulating and accountable to the public. The national, regional and local infrastructure for this needs to be debated. This infrastructure should fully recognise the skills involved in policy development, partnership work and community action rather than relate to a medical model of health.

Health promotion specialists are a group for whom these skills are core. On the one hand, the survival of this important body of expertise depends on its exponents' adaptability and versatility in working in different contexts. On the other, their identity as a coherent group depends on their ability to sustain professional networks, maintain core principles of practice in a range of organisational situations and gain recognition for doing so.

References

Chambers, T. (1999) Missing links. *Health Management,* August: 16–17.

Chief Medical Officer's Review of the Public Health Function in Scotland (2000) http://www.scotland.gov.uk

Department of Health (1998a) *Smoking Kills.* London: Stationery Office.

Department of Health (1998b) *The New NHS: Modern, Dependable.* London: Stationery Office.

Department of Health (1999a) *Saving Lives: Our Healthier Nation.* London: Stationery Office.

Department of Health (1999b) *Leadership for Health* (HSC 1999/192). London: Stationery Office.

Department of Health (1999c) *National Service Framework: Mental Health.* London: Stationery Office.

Department of Health (2000) *National Service Framework: Coronary Heart Disease.* London: Stationery Office.

Ewles, L. (1996) The impact of the NHS reforms on specialist health promotion in the NHS. In Scriven, A. and Orme, J. (eds) *Health Promotion: Professional Perspectives.* Basingstoke: Macmillan.

French, J. (1999) *The Growing Problem of Pay Comparability and Recruitment.* Internal paper. Society of Health Education and Promotion Specialists.

Funnell, R., Oldfield, K. and Speller, V. (1995) *Towards Healthier Alliances: A Tool for Planning, Evaluating and Developing Healthy Alliances.* London: HEA/Wessex Institute of Public Health Medicine.

Gillies, P. (1999) *Evidence Base 2000.* London: HEA.

Healthwork UK (2000) *Bulletin No 1: Specialist Standards in Public Health.* London: Healthwork UK.

Learmonth, A. and Watson, W. (1999) Constructing evidence based health promotion: perspectives from the field. *Critical Public Health,* 9: 4.

Miller, C. (1998) *Joint Action on Health Inequalities: The Policy Drivers for the Health Service and for Local Authorities*. London: HEA.

Milner, S. and French, J. (1997) *A Survey of Health Promotion Specialists in Relation to Purchasing and Providing Arrangements in England, Wales and Northern Ireland* (carried out in November 1996). Glasgow: Society of Health Education and Promotion Officers.

Robertson, W. and MacDonald, G. (2000) *Interim Report of a National Survey of Specialist Health Promotion Services in the NHS (November–December 1999), Carried Out in the Context of the 1997/98 NHS Reforms*. Birmingham: University of Central England, Birmingham.

Social Exclusion Unit (1999) *Teenage Pregnancy*. London: Stationery Office.

Social Exclusion Unit (2000) *National Strategy for Neighbourhood Renewal: A Framework for Consultation*. London: Cabinet Office.

Society of Health Education and Promotion Specialists (1999) *A Quality Framework*. Available from S. Maclennan, 64 Terregles Avenue, Glasgow, G41 4LX.

Society of Health Education and Promotion Specialists (2000) *Multidisciplinary Public Health: A Briefing and Discussion Paper*. Available from S. Maclennan, 64 Terregles Avenue, Glasgow, G41 4LX.

Speller, V., Learmonth, A. and Harrison, D. (1997) The search for evidence of effective health promotion. *British Medical Journal*, **7104**: 361–3.

Welsh Office (1998) *Strategic Framework (Better Health, Better Wales)*. Cardiff: National Assembly for Wales www.wales.gov.uk.

World Health Organization (1986) *The Ottawa Charter*. Geneva: WHO.

World Health Organization (1998) *Health Promotion Glossary*. WHO/HPR/HEP/98.1. Geneva: WHO.

CHAPTER 7

The Potential for Health Promotion in Hospital Nursing Practice

SUE LATTER

The recent policy emphasis on consumer participation in healthcare has taken place against a backdrop of change in the pattern of disease and a shift towards self-care and the management of illness and rehabilitation in the community. This has been combined with an increasing emphasis on a holistic model of health within nursing, incorporating psychological and social as well as physical dimensions. The result has been a recognition that nursing needs to move beyond its traditional function of caring for the sick and embrace an expanded role in health education and health promotion. This is reflected in strategic and policy documents spanning the past 15 years from the United Kingdom Central Council for Nursing, Midwifery and Health Visiting's (1986) proposals for nurse education to the recommendations outlined in the recent Department of Health policy document *Making a Difference: Strengthening the Nursing, Midwifery and Health Visiting Contribution to Healthcare* (DoH, 1999a).

While the health promotion function of nurses working in primary healthcare settings enjoys a long tradition, it is only latterly that this has been applied to nurses working in hospitals. The potential contribution of hospital-based nurses to health promotion has been ill defined, as evidenced by the dearth of literature and empirical work available in this area. Many of the concepts central to health promotion are more readily applicable to the community or primary care setting than to the hospital context. For example, the application of key health promotion activities in the hospital context, such as building healthy public policy, creating supportive environments and strengthening community action (WHO, 1986), is a challenging task.

In addition, values central to health promotion – collaboration, public participation and empowerment – do not sit easily with the tradition of hospital healthcare. The latter has been founded on a medical model approach to care, characterised by an orientation towards cure, treatment in the medical environment, a tendency to dismiss the patient's perspective and an expectation of the patient role as one that involves passivity, trust and a willingness to wait for medical help (Hart, 1991). These characteristics of the hospital environment need to be continually reassessed by healthcare professionals not only in the interests of ideologically and ethically sound practice, but also in the light of the clinical governance framework within which nurses and other healthcare professionals operate, that is, the requirement for clinically effective practice based on the best possible available evidence.

The vast number of hospital nurses, and their close and continuous contact with patients during an episode of heightened awareness of their health and illness, suggests that they have a powerful potential contribution to make to the health promotion movement. An exploration of the opportunities available for health promotion in hospital nursing practice follows below. Nurses' role as health educators with patients is first reviewed. This is followed by an analysis of nurses' potential contribution to collaborative work on health issues at a broader, health promotion level. Constraints that may militate against the achievement of this potential are also highlighted.

Hospital nurses as health educators

Currently, the focus of hospital nurses' practice usually revolves around care for the individual patient. An important element of their health promotion potential thus concerns the health education interactions in which they may engage with patients. Individual education comprises an element of health promotion, together with action at a broader structural or policy level (Macdonald and Bunton, 1992). This aspect of the hospital nurse's role in health promotion has historically been enacted in the form of patient education on disease management and structured information giving to patients in preparation for stressful events or procedures. There exists a substantial body of empirical evidence to suggest that these activities have a beneficial health outcome, such as reduced anxiety and an improved recovery rate. However, they have traditionally tended to be characterised by an emphasis on compliance and by didactic, standardised approaches. More recently, the need to adopt more individualised, patient-centred approaches, incorporating a recognition of the importance of self-efficacy beliefs and the wider barriers to taking health action, has been widely recognised (see, for example, van Ryn and Heaney, 1997; Norton, 1998).

Further aspects of hospital nurses' potential role in health education can be outlined by drawing on theoretical literature. Tones and Tilford (1994), for example, outline a model of health promotion that depicts an educational component referred to as critical consciousness raising. This refers to the idea that, through a health education encounter, individuals may be encouraged to think critically about their lives and circumstances, and the health educator may raise awareness of the wider factors that determine health choices. This may then lead to collective action at a community level, pressurising those with power to adopt more health-promoting policies.

Draper's (1983) analysis of types of health education information also indicates further areas that hospital nurses need to consider as part of their health education role. He outlines the provision of information on preventative health services, education about the environment and how this influences health, and education on the politics of health as a legitimate form of health education. One can suggest that there may be opportunities for hospital nurses to engage in dialogues of this nature with patients as part of their health promotion potential. A final strand to this health education role is highlighted by Downie et al.'s (1991) contention that health education not only involves communication activity with members of the community or general public (in this case patients), but is also aimed at professionals and those with power.

Research that enables definitive statements to be made about the extent to which nurses in hospitals enact elements of this health education role is scarce. However, research by the author (Latter, 1994) and by Macleod Clark et al. (1992) suggests that the reality falls short of the potential. Observation of nursing practice on wards employed as case studies revealed a minimal integration of health education into nurses' practice. There was a tendency for education to be nurse led, disease orientated and standardised, with a lack of evidence that nurses were engaging patients in dialogue about wider health issues or communicating with other professionals and policy makers about health promotion issues.

More recently, research into the nurse's role in educating patients on medication (Latter et al., 2000) highlighted that, in some clinical contexts, the potential for information giving and patient participation was not being fulfilled. In addition, the evidence base for effective interaction was neither recognised nor exploited by nurses. Possible reasons for this limited development of nurses' potential are discussed later in this chapter.

Expanding the health promotion role for hospital nurses

Current health promotion policies and health service changes necessitate a reconsideration of traditional patterns of hospital nursing work. That is, nurses' potential contribution to health promotion includes an involvement in activities over and above their bedside health education interactions with patients. Whereas these will remain an important element of their role, there is a need to embrace new ways of working that are consistent with health promotion concepts and principles. Nurses need to recognise and develop their potential role in the broader arena of health promotion in addition to their more traditional role as health educators. Creating environments that are supportive of health, encouraging community participation in health matters and helping to build healthy policies may all form part of the potential for health promotion in hospital nursing practice.

This will not, however, be achieved by all grades of nurse, or by nurses alone: there is a need to work in partnership with others across traditional boundaries. Recent UK health service legislation and policy may create opportunities for collaborative working. At a national level, the UK government has outlined the importance of this by recommending the need for healthy alliances, joint action and a better coordination of the range of departments and agencies in pursuit of the targets outlined in *Saving Lives: Our Healthier Nation* (DoH, 1999b). Naidoo and Wills (1994) propose that part of the contracts and service specifications produced by the purchasers of health services could include certain standards of health education and promotion, such as a smoke-free environment or the provision of healthy catering for National Health Service employees. The implication is that these standards will require collaboration between the various agencies involved, including nurses. The formation of alliances with other sectors, other professionals or voluntary groups requires a vision by hospital nurses of ways of working beyond the traditional boundaries of the bedside and of the ward itself.

Before considering the opportunities available for developing this aspect of hospital nursing practice, it is necessary to be clear about the contribution that this group of professionals can make to collaborative work for health. While it is evident that the responsibility for health promotion does not rest with the health sector alone, nurses nevertheless have a unique contribution to make to alliances created in the pursuit of promoting health. Their close and continuous contact with patients and their carers inevitably gives a detailed and holistic understanding of their physical, psychological and social needs, as well as of the extent to which these are met by current service provision. Hospital nurses are also in a position to identify particular patterns and trends in admission and can thus contribute their perspective to an assessment of local health needs as part of a public health approach. Nurses' specialised knowledge of health, the management of disease processes and the prevention of complications also means that they are well placed to contribute to education and awareness-raising exercises within the hospital or broader community.

Collaborative working within the hospital

Opportunities for collaborative working for health exist within the hospital environment as well as extending beyond its boundaries to the local community in which it is situated. Within the hospital, there is a need for nurses to engage with others in the process of creating and implementing policies that promote health. Examples of relevant policies include, as mentioned above, those set up to ensure smoke-free zones or those which promote healthy food choices for both patients and staff. Hospital-wide health promotion initiatives are recommended by McBride and Moorwood (1994) as being more effective than those involving isolated wards as they have the potential to be more cost-effective, encourage multi-disciplinary participation and allow the cross-fertilisation of ideas between staff from different patient areas. For example, a focus on the hospital as a health-promoting environment might involve nurses liaising with other disciplines within the hospital, such as occupational health and catering managers, as well as local authority environmental health officers and planners, the local media and lay members of the community.

In addition, patient and employer participation in the functioning of the hospital organisation is an important aspect of health promotion. Robinson and Hill (1998) suggest that one aspect of the work of a health-promoting nurse should be a contribution to supporting changes in resource provision, such as in dressings, members of staff or medication. These exemplify areas in which nurses can bring their perspective to bear in pursuit of policies that promote health within the hospital.

The establishment of patient or carer groups represents a further mechanism for promoting health in hospitals and may also provide the opportunity for nurses to collaborate with other agencies or disciplines. In mapping out the repertoire of health promotion, Beattie (1991) suggests that a 'personal counselling for health' approach may involve help provided through processes occurring within a group of peers with a group leader. Such groups may have a supportive and/or an educative function, and nurses may have a role as initiators, facilitators or occasional contributors, depending on the nature of the group itself.

With the trend towards a shorter admission period for patients, it becomes increasingly necessary to consider new ways of meeting patients' and carers' needs. The establishment of groups for patients or carers with similar needs, in either the pre-admission or the post-discharge period, represents one way forward. A successful example is cardiac rehabilitation groups for patients who have experienced a myocardial infarction or cardiac surgery. The nature of these vary widely, but they are often characterised by multi-disciplinary educational input from specialists such as dieticians, physiotherapists and counsellors, as well as from nurses. Nurses' insight into the experiences that patients are likely to encounter during their admission and their knowledge of the requirements of the rehabilitation process mean that they can make a valuable contribution to such groups.

Collaboration with the community

The potential for health promotion in hospital nursing practice also includes liaison and collaboration with agencies working to promote health in the community. Recent trends in healthcare have contributed to a breaking down of the boundaries that once established hospitals as discrete institutions isolated from the broader community. The hospital is a part of the community in which it is situated, and health promotion initiatives should be based on this principle. One way in which this might be achieved is through the Healthy Hospitals initiative, the hospital playing a role in local coalitions and strategies as part of the World Health Organization's Healthy Cities initiative. In addition, outreach or hospital-at-home teams and hospital–community liaison roles have developed in response to reduced admission periods, these providing opportunities for collaboration across traditional boundaries in relation to, for example, patient and carer information needs that support effective early discharge. The recent policy emphasis on consumer involvement in healthcare decision making and resource allocation also provides an important impetus for creating mechanisms for ensuring community participation in the priorities and functioning of the hospital healthcare system.

A further way in which hospital nurses might work collaboratively is by going out into the community and sharing their knowledge and expertise. Robinson and Hill (1998) highlight this as part of the work of a health-promoting nurse, suggesting that actions could include giving talks to self-help groups and raising awareness of a particular illness by supporting national campaigns. An example of this was highlighted by the author's investigation into the health promotion roles of hospital nurses (Latter, 1994). A ward sister working on a specialist ward for neuromuscular disorders liaised regularly with the local support group for those affected by multiple sclerosis and gave talks to interested members on aspects of disease management. She also spoke to local women's and church groups on various topics associated with neuromuscular disorders. This collaboration was two way in that volunteer workers from local support groups visited patients and carers on the ward who were in need of support.

However, the research highlighted that nurses' involvement in collaborative work for health is limited. With the exception of the example cited above, there was scant evidence of collaborative working away from direct caregiving at the bedside. From an interview sample of 132 ward sisters, only one or two isolated examples emerged. One ward sister reported formal liaison with a local health promotion officer and the hospital catering manager with a view to influencing the menu choices available in the hospital; another had been asked to join a multi-disciplinary health authority working party on nutrition policy. Although not focusing exclusively on hospital nurses, a study by Gott and O'Brien (1990a) revealed a similar picture. Their findings illustrated a nursing approach to health promotion orientated towards the provision of individualistic lifestyle advice and a lack of shared policies or broader action strategies for health promotion.

The way forward

If hospital nursing practice is to move forward towards the potential described here, a number of issues will need to be addressed. As a starting point, nurses require a sound understanding of the meaning of the concepts of health education and health promotion, as well as of their application to the hospital setting. Progress towards fulfilling this potential also dictates that nurses are equipped with relevant skills that enable them to take action. At the level of health education with individual patients, there must be a recognition of central concepts such as empowerment and holism, as well as the need for individualised approaches. Appropriate interpersonal skills are needed to operationalise these concepts in practice. Working with others to promote health beyond the bedside also requires an informed understanding of health promotion concepts and principles. When individuals are operating with different and conflicting personal models of health promotion, this can act as a barrier to effective communication (Cribb and Dines, 1993; Benson and Latter, 1998). Nurses will also need to be proficient in skills such as those outlined by Naidoo and Wills (1994): communication, participation in meetings, managing paperwork and time, and being and working in a group.

The author's research (Latter, 1994) highlighted that hospital nurses were operating with a very limited perception of health education and health promotion, one akin to an illness-orientated, individualistic approach. Findings indicated that there was generally a lack of recognition of the broader policy or structural aspect of health promotion, and none of those interviewed made reference to the principle of intersectoral collaboration as part of their understanding of health promotion. Opportunities are nevertheless available to address such deficits in understanding. Within nurse education, a central aim of the preregistration Project 2000 (UKCC, 1986) proposals was to equip nurses of the future for their role as health promoters, based on a sound understanding of health promotion theory. Qualified, practising nurses have also been able to update their knowledge and skills in health promotion through accessing post-registration programmes. Also, as the author has suggested elsewhere (Latter, 1998), there is some evidence to suggest that a more sophisticated understanding of health education and health promotion now permeates nurse education curricula than was originally the case in the early 1990s.

Education about health promotion knowledge and skills is, however, unlikely, by itself, to be sufficient to enable nurses to fulfil their potential in a hospital setting. Enacting the strategies outlined above will also necessitate a consideration of new ways of working over and above the historical focus on ward specialities and care delivered to individual patients. Grasping opportunities for collaboration and the forging of healthy alliances means working across ward and hospital boundaries that have been created as a consequence of a focus on illness as opposed to health promotion. As well as informal networking, organisational structures in the hospital setting need to be established and supported whereby multi-agency work on health promotion issues is possible. This might involve nurse management representation on multi-disciplinary or multi-agency health promotion committees or forums.

The current political emphasis on reducing waiting lists for hospital admissions creates both opportunities for and barriers to working in different ways. On the one hand, a shorter hospital stay means that hospital nurses are increasingly working with patients in a window of time when they are acutely ill and requiring technological expertise. This means prioritising the individualistic focus on bedside nursing at the expense of the collective approaches referred to above. Even this individualistic focus may preclude health education if the patient is too acutely ill to be receptive to information and dialogue about health. On the other hand, pre-admission assessments for surgical patients and early discharge support teams create new opportunities for both health education and collaborative working across professional and contextual boundaries.

All hospital nurses clearly require technical skills and those which facilitate empowering health education interactions, as well as the ability to apply these judiciously to the context and individual patients with whom they work. More senior grades of staff are more likely to have the confidence, experience and opportunity to work away from the bedside to create collaboration and influence policy as part of the broader health promotion potential referred to above. The recent creation of nurse consultant posts provides an important opportunity for the latter.

A final issue that will need to be addressed concerns the status and autonomy of nurses. If nurses are to empower patients as part of their health education role and work in collaboration with other key players in the promotion of health, it is essential that they are invested with the authority and autonomy to do so. In a key nursing text, Pearson (1988) suggests that autonomy for patients means autonomy for nurses because the nurse who is with the patient is otherwise powerless to allow the patient to carry out the decisions he or she makes. Tones (1993) also makes this connection clear. He states that any policy designed to achieve a health-promoting hospital should not overlook the fact that a hospital comprises a community of both patients and staff. Its aim should therefore be to empower not only patients, but also staff.

Status and authority to influence organisational decisions are also a prerequisite for successful collaborative ventures with other groups or agencies involved in health promotion. Historically, nurses have not enjoyed such status or authority, either individually or collectively. As Gott and O'Brien (1990b) have highlighted, the nursing profession has had near-universal subordinate status vis-à-vis other professions and interests, and nurses have been afforded little authority or control in a healthcare system dominated by the priorities of its superordinate allied professions. More recently, the drive to create accessible and patient-focused healthcare has led to the creation of more autonomous roles for nurses, as evidenced, for example, by NHS Direct and walk-in centres. As such trends in health service policy and practice have begun to erode traditional role boundaries, the 'subordinate' status of nurses may arguably give way to a clearer recognition of their expertise on the part of both other professionals and the public.

Nurse education has a role to play in preparing nurses for new roles and responsibilities, and Tones' (1993) suggestion that assertiveness training should form part of the nurse education curriculum to support their health promotion function and contribute to their sense of professional identity is relevant here. Perhaps what are also required are systems of nurse education that foster empowerment and a philosophy of practice that values the centrality of nursing expertise, as well as systems of care organisation that allow individual nurses the power to make decisions and act on them.

To conclude, nursing in the 21st century must re-evaluate traditional methods of delivering healthcare and create new ways of working that are congruent with current health trends and policy changes. The potential for health promotion in hospital nursing practice includes both health education with individual patients and working across professional boundaries to collaborate with others in the spirit of health promotion. Nurses need education in health promotion knowledge and skills, as well as organisational structures within the hospital, to enable collaborative working on health issues. Increased status and autonomy for the nursing profession is also needed in order that nurses can fulfil their health promotion potential.

References

Beattie, A. (1991) Knowledge and control in health promotion: a test case for social policy and social theory. In Gabe, J., Calnan, M. and Bury, M. (eds) *The Sociology of the Health Service*. London: Routledge.

Benson, A. and Latter, S. (1998) The influence of a research study on the integration of health promotion and interpersonal skills within nursing curricula. *Journal of Advanced Nursing*, **27**: 100–7.

Cribb, A. and Dines, A. (1993) What is health promotion? In Dines, A. and Cribb, A. (eds) *Health Promotion: Concepts and Practice*. Oxford: Blackwell Scientific.

Department of Health (1999a) *Making a Difference*. London: Stationery Office.

Department of Health (1999b) *Saving Lives: Our Healthier Nation*. London: Stationery Office.

Downie, R.S, Fyfe, C. and Tannahill, A. (1991) *Health Promotion: Models and Values* (revised edn). Oxford: Oxford Medical Publications.

Draper, P. (1983) Tackling the disease of ignorance. *Self-Health*, **1**: 23–5.

Gott, M. and O'Brien, M. (1990a) Practice and the prospect for change. *Nursing Standard*, **10**(5): 30–2.

Gott, M. and O'Brien, M. (1990b) *The Role of the Nurse in Health Promotion: Policies, Perspectives and Practice*. Report of a two-year research project funded by the Department of Health/Department of Health and Social Welfare. Milton Keynes: Open University.

Hart, N. (1991) *The Sociology of Health and Medicine*. Ormskirk: Causeway Press.

Latter, S. (1994) Health education and health promotion: perceptions and practice of nurses in acute care settings. Unpublished PhD thesis, King's College, University of London.

Latter, S. (1998) Nursing, health education and health promotion: lessons learned, progress made and challenges ahead. *Health Education Research*, **13**(2): i–v.

Latter, S., Yerrell, P, Rycroft-Malone, J. and Shaw, D. (2000) *Nursing and Medication Education: The Preparation and Role of Nurses in Patients', Clients' and Carers' Medication Education*. Final Report. London: ENB.

Macleod Clark, J., Wilson-Barnett, J., Latter, S. and Maben, J. (1992) *Health Education and Health Promotion in Nursing: A Study of Practice in Acute Areas*. Report of a two-tier research project funded by the Department of Health/Department of Nursing Studies. London: King's College, University of London.

McBride, A. and Moorwood, Z. (1994) The hospital health promotion facilitator: an evaluation. *Journal of Clinical Nursing*, **3**: 355–9.

Macdonald, G. and Bunton, R. (1992) Health promotion: discipline or disciplines? In Bunton, R. and Macdonald, G. (eds) *Health Promotion: Disciplines and Diversity*. London: Routledge.

Naidoo, J. and Wills, J. (1994) *Health Promotion: Foundations for Practice*. London: Baillière Tindall.

Norton, L. (1998) Health promotion and health education: what role should the nurse adopt in practice? *Journal of Advanced Nursing*, **28**(6): 1269–75.

Pearson, A. (ed.) (1988) *Primary Nursing: Nursing in the Burford and Oxford Nursing Development Units*. London: Croom Helm.

Robinson, S. and Hill, Y. (1998) The health promoting nurse. *Journal of Clinical Nursing*, **7**: 232–8.

Tones, K. (1993) The theory of health promotion: implications for nursing. In Wilson-Barnett, J. and Macleod Clark, J. (eds) *Research in Health Promotion and Nursing*. Basingstoke: Macmillan.

Tones, K. and Tilford, S. (1994) *Health Education: Effectiveness, Efficiency and Equity*. London: Chapman & Hall.

United Kingdom Central Council for Nursing, Midwifery and Health Visiting (1986) *Project 2000*. London: UKCC.

van Ryn, M. and Heaney, C.A. (1997) Developing effective helping relationships in health education practice. *Health Education and Behaviour*, **24**(6): 683–702.

World Health Organization (1986) *Ottawa Charter for Health Promotion*. Ottowa: WHO.

PART III

LOCAL AUTHORITIES

INTRODUCED AND EDITED BY JUDY ORME

The contribution of local authorities to public health has become increasingly visible in recent policy documentation. Their breadth of responsibility for public services demonstrates their centrality to improving health, and their potential for collaboration is enormous. This includes collaboration across the health and social care interface, a key involvement in Health Improvement Programmes (HImPs) and the membership of Primary Care Groups.

The emphasis on improving the social, economic and environmental well-being of their communities to incorporate the production of community plans is a clear demonstration of the additional potential for joint planning and working over and above HImP, Health Action Zone and Healthy City partnerships.

The three chapters in this section clearly demonstrate the important roles that local authorities play in promoting health. The discussion covers environmental health and social services, followed by an overview of the promotion of physical activity in the local authority setting.

The first chapter, written by Peter Allen, acknowledges that the contribution of environmental health to the public health agenda is well documented. He argues, however, that the visibility of the potential capacity and capability of environmental health in collaborative working to promote health needs to be strengthened. This chapter helps to increase this visibility by demonstrating the multi-faceted contribution of the environmental health agenda.

Linda Jones and Wendy Rose, in Chapter 9, reflect on the potential for promoting health in the very pressured realm of social services provision. They argue that government policy has in recent years supported a comprehensive approach to health promotion that focuses first on prevention and early intervention to avoid crises, second on appropriate information and support to clients, and third on collaborative working that acknowledges the interrelatedness of health and social care goals. This is all set against a background of pressure on resources and demand, and continuing organisational turbulence. The authors raise key issues surrounding the potential and dilemmas that this setting presents for health promotion.

Robin Ireland's chapter discusses the challenges of working in partnership to develop sport and transport policies that are accessible, appropriate and available at local level, and uncovers a range of dilemmas. The need to ensure that the social context of people's lives remains a central driving force for these developments is paramount. This chapter concludes this section by discussing these issues and gives insight into the practicalities of this work using many national and local examples.

CHAPTER 8

Health Promotion, Environmental Health and Local Authorities

PETER ALLEN

Saving Lives: Our Healthier Nation (DoH, 1999), like its predecessor *The Health of the Nation* (DoH, 1992), recognises that local authorities are responsible for a wide range of public services, many of which are linked with the strategy set out in the White Paper. These responsibilities include education, environmental control, environmental health and food safety, transport, housing and social services. This chapter looks at what local authorities can do to advance health in particular through their environmental health officers (EHOs).

The difference between local government authorities and health authorities

There is a significant difference between local government authorities and health authorities. In health authorities, accountability is predominantly upwards to the Secretary of State, with enormous powers to make key appointments and make financial resources available. On the other hand, accountability in local government is predominantly downward to local people. Healthy alliances between the two types of authority are crucial if health is to be promoted effectively. If a health authority tries to work in isolation with regard to health promotion, without linking with the local authority, it foregoes the unique relationship that exists between the town hall and its local people. Furthermore, if a local authority distances itself from the health authority, it misses out on the wider perspective, particularly the expertise and relevant experience.

Another important point that needs to be made is that local authorities, like health authorities, possess a dynamic structure that is subject to change. The present situation in local government is something of a mishmash, with some parts having a two-tier system continuing at county and district level, whereas other county councils and district councils have given way to 'unitary' councils. Thus, in the former, important health promotion services such as social services and education are in one local authority – a county council – and other equally important health promotion services such as housing, leisure and environmental health lie in another – a district council. In the latter, the new unitary councils, all the functions are within the same authorities, but how they are arranged can vary. In some authorities, various housing functions are outsourced, whereas in others they are not. It can be confusing to even the keenest observer let alone the public. This should not, however, discourage health promotion practitioners. It is simply making clear that we need to take the concept of health partnerships to a deeper level and see the need for its application not just between local authorities and health authorities and others but between local authorities and between the different professionals that make up local government.

Role models

Before examining environmental health services, which is the main focus of this chapter, it is worth making one further point. In England and Wales, there are over 400 local authorities with nearly two and half million employees. In terms of the employment market, this is a substantial segment. If local authorities take action to introduce effective health policies, they can not only provide their internal community with an opportunity for better health, but also provide a role model for local commerce and industry. Many have followed this approach on specific health promotion issues.

The Institution of Environmental Health Officers carried out a survey to establish the situation with regard to smoking. They found that 85 per cent of local authorities that responded had in fact established non-smoking policies. To help local authorities, the Institute, along with the Health Education Authority (HEA), has published *Guidelines for Smoking Policies in Local Authorities* (IEHO, 1993). This booklet contains a step-by-step guide as well as much other useful information. Local authorities can therefore act as local role models in a wide range of health aspects from balanced alcohol policies to good green practice.

The contribution of local authority environmental health services to health promotion

There was a time when it was argued that health promotion and enforcement were different entities, but 'health promotion' is now increasingly being seen as an umbrella term to cover all interventions that promote health, including enforcement. As Tones (1990) points out, health promotion incorporates all measures deliberately designed to promote health and handle disease.

The environmental health enforcement duties of local authorities are set out in legislation and cover:

- food inspection and food hygiene and safety;
- housing standards;
- health and safety at work and during recreation;
- environmental protection, including statutory nuisances;
- communicable disease prevention and control;
- licensing;
- drinking water surveillance;
- refuse collection and street cleansing;
- pest control.

A detailed description of these duties is set out in the EHO's handbook (Bassett, 1999). However, as far as health promotion is concerned, what needs to be noted is that the above mandatory enforcement duties are vital if health is to be advanced. People, for example, need sound and adequate housing. It is inappropriate simply to provide a first-class primary healthcare service and new hospitals if adequate and suitable housing is not provided. Nor does it make sense in economic terms. Illness caused by poor housing is estimated to cost the NHS £2 billion a year (Standing Conference on Public Health, 1994). This has obvious implications for our limited National Health Service resources.

Discretionary powers

EHOs also have an extensive range of discretionary powers (see, for example, those detailed in section 54 of the Public Health Act 1964 and the Home Safety Act of 1961. These discretionary powers can make a significant contribution to health promotion. In recent years, work carried out under these sections has covered such topics as HIV/AIDS, alcohol and drug addiction, nutrition, women's health, men's health, heating and energy advice, occupational health, health aspects of poverty, greening (environmental enhancement), health grants to voluntary organisations and of course the range of varied activities covered by home safety.

An example of how a local authority can, through its discretionary powers, promote health can be seen in the Oxford Airwatch Partnership Project. In the early 1990s, Oxford City Council was faced with growing concern about ill health caused by traffic. It was also, like other local authorities, faced with ambivalent standards. First there was pollution, but no money to monitor the effects. (The government had funded only a handful of monitoring stations, mostly at background sites.) Second, there appeared to be no real commitment on behalf of the government to secure car-free cities and locally managed public transport systems: the policy of bus deregulation had been left largely to market determination.

The first step was to convince the local council that traffic pollution was a priority. This presented difficulties because there was no money to fund the initial monitoring. The EHOs decided to enter the barter economy. They located a reputable company that was just starting to enter the local authority monitoring market. In return for a free six-month loan of equipment, the EHOs gave the company a prime city centre site plus a place in their forward plan to develop a European initiative to highlight the above concerns.

Within six months, the local council was, thanks to the results of the monitoring, convinced that they did have a traffic pollution problem, and, to their credit, they gave full backing under their discretionary powers to move forward with the Airwatch Partnership Project. The main partners in the project are set out in Figure 8.1.

Although it is still in its initial stages, the partnership is already bearing fruit. Bonn is a car-free city, Lieden has developed a theoretical model of pollution forecasts, Grenoble has developed, to a high degree, central and local planning, and Oxford has its park and ride scheme. All these things are being shared to great benefit, as is the local research on health and traffic. The point for health promotion practitioners is that the environmental health discretionary powers of local authorities can contribute to promoting health in a very real way.

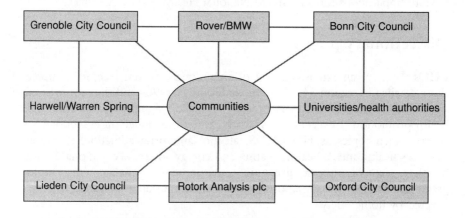

Figure 8.1   Partners in the Airwatch Partnership Project

Campaigns and projects

It is, perhaps, helpful in the context of this book to look at a number of local campaigns and projects in which EHOs work in health promotion partnership with the health authority, commerce and industry.

Restaurants, cafés and hotels are regularly inspected by EHOs under the Food Safety Act, so these officers are in a strong position to encourage above statutory minimum standards. The HEA's Heartbeat Award scheme, introduced jointly by the HEA and individual local authorities, has provided a means of promoting and establishing healthy eating options and no smoking areas in catering premises. Some local authorities have gone further and established their own food awards for the catering industry, which enhance the Heartbeat standard and encourage additional health facilities such as baby-changing accommodation and the provision of non-alcoholic drink.

Commercial premises other than catering premises can also be encouraged in a similar fashion. One local authority introduced, jointly with their health authority, a health award. In order to attain the award, a company had to comply completely with the Health and Safety at Work Act and in addition commit itself to three approved green policies and three approved healthy lifestyle policies.

By setting up a good landlord or (to be politically correct) good landperson award, a number of local authorities are promoting health by encouraging the former to see their business as a positive health contribution to the local community.

Participation in local campaigns and projects is laudable, but they are more effective when interacting with a national campaign. Such central organisations as the Health Development Agency or the Department of Health can set the national agenda by attracting media coverage and a high profile for their national figures. They can also provide expertise to give a campaign firm direction. Add to this the local authority's local network and there is productive synergy.

So far in this chapter, we have looked at health promotion in terms of health, that is, health in its broadest terms, which includes the environment. In the last 15 years, however, we have also seen a separate movement emerging, the environmental movement. This reached its zenith in 1992 at the United Nations Conference on environment and development (the Earth Summit), held in Rio de Janeiro, Brazil. Over 150 nations, including the UK, endorsed a 500-page document, Agenda 21, which set out how both developed and developing countries could work towards sustainable development (United Nations, 1992). This has been nearly summarised in a booklet by the then Local Government Management Board (LGMB, 1993).

Agenda 21 singles out local government as having a special role, two-thirds of the actions in Agenda 21 requiring the active involvement of local authorities. Chapter 28 of Agenda 21 called on them to begin local Agenda 21 processes – partnerships for sustainable development at a local level – by 1996. (By the end of 1996, roughly three-quarters of them had published action plans.) The government has now relaunched the strategy.

There was initially an element of 'tribalism' between the health and environmental movements. It was possible, for example, to go to the World Health Organization Healthy City conferences and search in vain for the environmental input, or in contrast to review the papers of car-free city conferences only to discover that health was very much an also-ran. In recent years, shared membership, fresh vision and joint campaigning has done much to blur the boundaries between the two movements. EHOs with a foot in both the environmental and health camps, as well as recent experience of helping to advance 'Health for All', have been well placed locally to focus the two movements. Indeed, a number of local authorities have transformed their health promotion units into health and environmental promotion units to capitalise on the synergy that comes when these two powerful movements work together.

Conclusion

Local authorities can, through their EHOs, make an important contribution to health promotion. Since 1974, when the medical officer was relocated in the health authority, the EHO has been seen as the local authority's lead officer on health matters. It is, however, now recognised that to promote health effectively, professionals need to work on a collaborative basis rather than as independent experts. Health is indeed everybody's business, and if anyone should lead, it should be the community. It is now acknowledged that local government departments such as personnel, education, social services and leisure also have a key role in health promotion. What parts they have to play will be discussed later in this book.

References

Bassett, W.H. (1999) *Clay's Handbook of Environmental Health* (18th edn). London: Chapman & Hall.

Department of Health (1992) *The Health of the Nation*. London: HMSO.

Department of Health (1999) *Saving Lives: Our Healthier Nation*. London: Stationery Office.

Institute of Environmental Health Officers (1993) *Guidance to Local Authorities on Smoking Policies*. London: IEHO.

Local Government Management Board (1993) *Local Agenda 21: Principles and Process: a Step by Step Guide*. London: Local Government Management Board.

Standing Conference on Public Health (1994) *A National Strategy for Housing*. London: SCPH.

Tones, K. (1990) Why theorise: ideology in health education. *Health Education Journal*, **49**: 1.

United Nations (1992) *Earth Summit. Agenda 21: The United Nations Programme of Action from Rio*. New York: UN Department of Information.

CHAPTER 9

Social Services and Health Promotion: Towards Independence and Empowerment

LINDA JONES AND WENDY ROSE

Social services have a growing workload and a budget of nearly £9,500 million, rising to £12,208 million in 2003–04. Social service departments know of 300,000–400,000 children in need, of whom 53,000 are in some type of statutory care and 32,000 are on Child Protection Registers (DoH, 1999a). Around 100,000 people, including older people and those with physical disabilities, learning disabilities and mental health problems, are being supported by social services in local authority, voluntary or private residential homes (Central Statistical Office, 1998). Many thousands of families are visited by social workers each year and during the 1990s home care services expanded significantly to service nearly half a million households.

This breadth of provision, delivered in a range of intimate and formal settings, indicates that social services have considerable potential to promote people's health. In looking at their role, however, it is important to start off with an explicit recognition of their limitations. Unlike schools or primary healthcare services, these departments are not universal providers of services: the majority of citizens go through life without direct contact with them. Social services could not be expected to provide mass health promotion in the way that primary healthcare might aim to do. However, since they work with many of the most vulnerable, frail and socially disadvantaged people in society, they have a potentially strategic role in any overall health promotion strategy. This has been increasingly recognised in government policy in the UK, especially since 1997.

Linking social services to health promotion goals

Many of the goals established for health promotion are relevant to the work of social services. The Ottawa Charter (WHO, 1986) emphasised the need

95

to create supportive environments, strengthen community action and develop personal skills so that people had the resources to influence and improve their health. *Health 21* (WHO, 1998), which set new targets for the European region, re-stated Health for All goals in terms of empowering people to realise their potential by linking better health to economic and social development. The UK health promotion strategies of the late 1990s focused more explicitly on tackling social inequality and social exclusion through fostering participation, community development and interagency partnerships. In England, this emphasis was fuelled by the Independent Inquiry into Inequalities in Health, led by Sir Donald Acheson (DoH, 1998a). This identified 'unacceptable inequalities' in health and called for priority action to reduce income inequality and help families with children.

Social services already engage in health promotion activity by protecting their clients and working to develop their skills for living. In recent years, however, a more comprehensive approach to health promotion has begun to be developed. The focus of this is threefold: prevention and early intervention to avoid crises; health education, offering appropriate information and support to clients; and building healthy alliances that acknowledge the interrelatedness of social and healthcare goals. After discussing the focus of social services, we draw attention to opportunities and new initiatives, and consider how this strategic approach is being developed with different client groups.

Social services: priorities and pressures

In spite of increasing interest in prevention and health promotion in the 1990s, there was also growing pressure on social services to concentrate their efforts and resources at the more intensive end of the care spectrum, on those already in crisis. Several important factors influenced this development. A growing demand for services outstripped the supply of resources. This was most evident with the rising population of frail elderly people. Unemployment also remained a significant feature: in 1997, 3 million working-age people had been dependent on benefits for over two years (DSS, 1999).

Second, there was a continued upheaval associated with the restructuring of services and the creation in social services departments of commissioner and provider wings. National Health Service (NHS) reforms increased the demand for social services. The dramatic fall in the number of long-stay hospital geriatric beds, for example, had a profound impact upon the type and level of home care services required. These upheavals were compounded by problems of recruiting and retaining social services staff in what was becoming an ageing workforce (DoH, 1998b).

Finally, specific government legislation, such as the Mental Health Act 1983 and the Children Act 1989, as well as their sometimes legalistic and defensive interpretations by social services, resulted in an overconcentration on those deemed to be most at risk, particularly children. There seemed at times to be an almost exclusive concentration on protection at the expense of providing services to families whose children were in need but not at immediate risk of significant harm (Audit Commission, 1994).

The changing context of health promotion

The health categorisation of primary, secondary and tertiary prevention can provide a useful starting point for conceptualising social care interventions (Parker, 1980; Hardiker et al., 1991, 1999). Whereas primary prevention is aimed at the wider population, secondary prevention focuses on high risk and tertiary prevention on mitigating the damaging effects of breakdown by remedial interventions and on ensuring that the problem does not recur (Macdonald, 2000). Within a defensive culture, there is little chance of health promotion work gaining ground in social services departments. In a more open and accountable culture, however, social services objectives can be aligned more closely with health promotion objectives, focusing not just on tertiary interventions, but also on primary and secondary measures to protect and enhance quality of life.

Until the late 1990s, it could be claimed that primary prevention in social care, once prominent in the community development projects of the 1960s and characterised as 'influencing the social-structural origins of personal troubles', largely belonged in the category of abandoned ambitions (Fuller, 1992). *Modernising Social Services* and *Partnerships in Action* (DoH, 1998b, c) signalled a change of priorities, emphasising the importance of promoting user independence through better preventive services. Initiatives such as Sure Start, Health Improvement Programmes and Health Action Zones, together with the setting up of new agencies such as the Social Exclusion Unit, brought a re-awakening of interest in community-based approaches. These were aimed at encouraging interagency working to transform areas of deprivation, enhancing choice and quality of life, and providing services to people at risk of exclusion from mainstream society. The sections that follow explore the impact of changing priorities for different client groups.

Children and families

Preventive work with children and families involves a widening of priorities so that child protection, focused on investigating cases of physical and sexual abuse, is complemented and underpinned by a broader network of services that support children in need and their families before breakdown and violence occur. This might involve, for example, plans to stimulate networks of support and self-reliance, offer simple practical services such as occasional respite during a family crisis or provide guidance through the benefits maze.

By the late 1990s, this wider vision for children and families was beginning to become embedded in policy and practice. In the aftermath of the Children Act 1989, the reactive policing of abuse had resulted in some needy families receiving fewer services (Aldgate, cited in Cervi, 1994). This approach was questioned by the Department of Health (DoH), which argued that:

> the primary focus of a social services department is not to find out whether a child has been abused or a criminal offence has occurred. Have we strayed from the notion of a social worker making inquiries and visiting a family at home to see if she or he can be helpful? (Rose, cited in Stone, 1994: 16)

Working Together to Safeguard Children (DoH/Home Office/DfEE, 1999) developed this view, promoting the earlier identification of need and a more balanced approach to the provision of services so that child protection was seen as one part of a wider provision for children in need. The subsequent guidance (DoH et al., 2000) argued that rather than focusing too narrowly on alleged incidences of neglect or abuse, agencies should be taking a wider view of the overall needs of children and their families. It would often be more effective to provide services and support to multiply disadvantaged families when problems first presented rather than waiting for difficulties to escalate into abuse. The Quality Protects programme (DoH, 1998d) set objectives and targets for local authorities to improve services for children in need and in care.

The overall objective was to promote equality of opportunity for all children, allowing them to fulfil their potential at school, in the labour market and as citizens. This involved creating environments in which children could flourish and their physical and mental health and well-being, and personal development, could be safeguarded.

Particular initiatives, for example the Social Exclusion Unit's work on teenage pregnancy (SEU, 1999), were developed to support this wider goal. This highlighted the poorer life and health chances of teenage mothers and launched a 10-year programme to improve support and education for young people. Social services were seen as playing a critical role in ensuring that sound advice was available on sex, contraception and sexual health, and they were set specific and measurable objectives to secure 'maximum life chance benefits from educational opportunities, healthcare and social care' (DoH, 1999d: 12) for groups such as looked after children. There was an expectation that local authorities and health authorities would 'agree the most appropriate set of health indicators in their communities, to which the work of social services departments contributes' (DoH, 1999c: 13).

Looked after children

In addition, social services have a particular responsibility and a unique opportunity to promote the health of children who come into public care.

These children are often among the most damaged and vulnerable of their generation, survivors of family breakdown, physical violence, neglect and sexual abuse. Guidance aimed at social services and health authorities has emphasised the opportunities to promote health for looked after children and the role that properly integrated services can have in reducing social exclusion (DoH, 2000).

Sexual health advice is a major priority (SEU, 1999), together with action on smoking. The White Paper *Smoking Kills* (DoH, 1998e) emphasised the need to deter young people from taking up smoking. DoH (1994) guidelines on smoking and alcohol consumption in residential homes advised that no child under 16 years of age should smoke and that staff and visitors should not smoke in front of children. Although desirable in health education terms, this proved difficult to enforce in residential homes, where cigarettes had become part of a reward system (Siddall, 1994).

Skills for independent living are also needed. Young people leaving local authority care constitute one of the groups most likely to become homeless (Boulton, 1993; Valios, 1999). Most looked after young people have been taught few skills and have found it difficult to cook, budget or manage the benefits system. Acknowledging this, DoH guidance (DoH, 2000) urged local authorities to set up advice and support systems and to develop the capacity of carers to support health promotion. In response, examples of good practice are emerging. These include Signpost, a multi-agency project in Wakefield, which offers housing and advice to young people leaving care (Valios, 1999); Barnsley social services are helping to fund health advice to carers and young people on health promotion issues such as safer sex, healthy living and taking exercise (DoH, 2000).

Services for older people

Promoting independence was an important theme in *Modernising Social Services* (DoH, 1998b), which envisaged not only improved preventive services, but also the extension of direct payments to people over 65 to buy care services for themselves and the provision of better support for their carers. Social services were urged to 'enable people to do things for themselves for as long as possible in their own homes' (p. 11), and to develop joint action plans with health authorities for prevention. In 1999, £100 million was provided over three years to stimulate support for people most at risk of losing their independence (Thompson, 2000). Since the early 1990s, therefore, home care services have expanded considerably. By 1998, local authorities purchased or provided 135 million hours of home care for 447,000 households, compared with 88 million hours in 1992. The focus shifted from home help, with its emphasis on cleaning and mechanical tasks, to home care, with its focus on personal as well as home care, as well as from direct provision by local authorities to contract provision.

The extension of the philosophy of primary prevention to older people, set out in *Modernising Social Services*, could bring considerable health gain if it were systematically pursued. Social services have direct contact with many thousands of older people through home care and meals-on-wheels services. Whether these services are provided directly or arranged on a contract basis by a voluntary agency or a private firm, there is a real opportunity to ensure that there is a health dimension to this work. Home carers often have considerable (unused) knowledge and understanding of the needs of their clients (Evers et al., 1994). They could offer not only information, for example on winter warmth campaigns, domestic accidents and access to services, but also much more of a link between clients and health and social services professionals. Tinker (1990) commented that the extension of home care services provided the context within which such proactive work could take place.

In the early 1990s, there was evidence that local authorities were so busy attempting to meet the rising demands for home care that they did not sufficiently evaluate their provision (Hoyes et al., 1994). By the end of the decade, it was budgetary constraint rather than demand that was threatening quality. The assumption that home care would be a cheaper option, which had driven much government thinking in this area, remained unproven. The consequence was 'that contracts between councils and the independent sector are now in danger merely of emphasising the supply of more services for the same money' (Thompson, 2000: 21). This may mean that promoting health remains a marginal activity.

In addition, the necessity of charging for services had meant that home care did not always reach those most in need (Becker, 1997), whereas NHS-provided services were free at the point of use. *Modernising Health and Social Services* (DoH, 1998f) announced plans to end this anomaly and bridge the divide between health and social care. The main steps were the introduction of pooled budgets, the integrated commissioning of health and social care within a locality and direct provision of a range of services, all of which could raise health promotion higher up the agenda.

Setting national standards for home care may also help to raise the quality of service, enforce health and safety standards, and strengthen health promotion work (Thompson, 2000). Key steps would be to target home care organisers and paid carers so that their role in home care could be extended to include systematic health advice and support. Training and support for informal carers on, for example, lifting techniques, first aid and diet could also feature on this wider agenda. Over six million people are currently caring for a relative or friend at home, and there is a need for practical as well as emotional support (Bibbings, 1994).

People with special needs

Most aspects of social services work relating to people with special needs have health promotion dimensions. For example, day care services provided for people with physical or learning disabilities, or mental health problems, sustain their general welfare and well-being and offer a vital break for carers. The assessment of needs and the provision for equipment and adaptations to enable people to continue living in their own homes is a vital service benefiting tens of thousands of people each year. It also has a strong health promotion dimension, offering people choice and independence.

The government agenda of the late 1990s, set out in *Modernising Social Services*, was directed towards promoting independence for people with special needs, including encouragement to enter paid employment and improved support for those with mental health problems. Interagency cooperation was seen as a key part of improved prevention. *Partnerships in Action* (DoH, 1998c: 15) stated that:

> the social care workforce will increasingly undertake joint working, particularly in areas such as mental health, drugs and alcohol, child abuse and learning disabilities.

Lack of resources, which has influenced progress on home care and day care provision, impacts on assessment as well. Since departments are bound under law to provide the full range of resources once needs have been demonstrated, social workers have tended to make a conservative estimate of need in case they are unable to meet it. By 1996, day care places, over 80 per cent of which were provided by the private sector, were increasingly being restricted (Drakeford, 2000). In addition, clients with less severe problems were being overlooked altogether. *Modernising Social Services* recognised this problem and the disadvantages of later, crisis intervention 'for the individual, the social services, the NHS and the taxpayer' (DoH, 1998b: 21). Bridging the Gap, a joint agency project involving local authorities and health authorities in London, has demonstrated how earlier intervention can save resources and protect health. This outreach service assesses and supports people with borderline learning difficulties, thus helping to prevent expensive admissions as well as combating social exclusion (Thompson, 2000).

The health dimension is probably most evident in the arena of mental health. Here, social work has a key role in counselling, support and advice, helping with specific mental health problems and arranging for specific medical and nursing services. In the mid-1990s, Tudor (1996: 167) lamented the lack of a mental health promotion policy at national level and the failure of community care for mental health service users, 'sacrificed on the ideological altar of the free market economy'. While mental health is still focused on policies to combat mental illness, the Labour administration did take steps to reverse the chronic underfunding of public services and to develop assertive services, additional secure units and 24-hour outreach teams in the community (Drakeford, 2000). Evidence so far suggests that sensitively organised assertive outreach work can offer early intervention and prevent at-risk people from being re-admitted (Dutt, 2000). Wilson and Francis (1997), investigating the provision of services to black mental health service users, noted that the success of outreach teams depended on recruiting suitably experienced staff with a more holistic and critical approach and a willingness to address the concerns of black people.

Interagency working

Effective interagency working lies at the heart of improving health outcome for vulnerable populations, yet it is notoriously difficult to achieve. As Hudson points out, failure in interagency collaboration highlighted in public inquiries is often followed by an exhortation to do more of it:

> Although the problems created by fragmentation are now more widely recognised, the reality is that policies have tended to be half-hearted and achievements are sometimes negligible. There is a paradox here, with collaboration seen as both problem and solution – failure to work together is the problem; therefore the solution is to work together better! (Hudson, 2000: 253)

Interagency work is essentially about human relationships, whether at a strategic planning level or in practice between front-line staff from different agencies. There is considerable scope for social services staff to liaise and network more effectively with doctors and community health staff in primary healthcare teams. Unified commissioning, pooled funding and new Primary Care Groups and Primary Care Trusts should speed up the development of multi-disciplinary teams delivering more coherent and coordinated services.

The health work–social work divide still, however, exists, professional training and occupational culture imbuing these services with attitudes and values that are difficult to change (Dalley, 1993). As long as the experience of professional working reinforces tribal loyalties, workers are likely to split along specialist professional lines when hard decisions have to be made. Such cleavages need to be recognised and tackled if health and social services are to work together to meet clients' health promotion needs.

Notwithstanding this, there has been a significant shift since the mid-1990s towards making the role of social services in health promotion more explicit. Government policy, in terms of restructuring, reports and guidance, has played a lead role in this. The challenges to social services remain considerable and involve improving coordination in policy and planning with health authorities at all levels. Holistic assessments of need by skilled practitioners, with access to appropriate specialist health advice and services, should be complemented by a more innovative, imaginative development of services, particularly in partnership with the voluntary sector. Social services will need to reappraise priorities to increase the capacity for early intervention and put more emphasis on effective staff training on the potential and importance of health and health promotion. Amidst the current pressure on resources and demand, and in the context of continuing organisational turbulence, it is unclear how far social services will be able to respond to these challenges.

References

Audit Commission (1994) *Seen But Not Heard*. London, HMSO.

Becker, S. (1997) *Responding to Poverty: The Politics of Cash and Care*. London: Longman.

Bibbings, A. (1994) Carers and professionals – the carer's viewpoint. In Leathard, A. (ed.) *Going Inter-Professional*. London: Routledge.

Boulton, 1. (1993) Youth homelessness and health care. In Fisher, K. and Collins, J. (eds) *Homelessness and Health Care*. London: Longman.

Central Statistical Office (1998) *Social Trends* (vol. 28). London: HMSO.

Cervi, R. (1994) Real lives. *Community Care*, (20 January): 16–17.

Dalley, G. (1993) Professional ideology or organisational tribalism? The health work–social work divide. In Walmsley, J., Reynolds, J., Shakespeare, P. and Wolfe, R. (eds) *Health, Welfare and Practice*. London: Sage.

Department of Health (1994) *Guidelines on Smoking and Alcohol Consumption in Residential Care Establishments*. London: HMSO.

Department of Health (1998a) *Independent Inquiry into Inequalities in Health*. London: Stationery Office.

Department of Health (1998b) *Modernising Social Services*. London: Stationery Office.

Department of Health (1998c) *Partnerships in Action: New Opportunities for Joint Working between Health and Social Services*. London: Stationery Office.

Department of Health (1998d) *The Quality Protects Programme* LAC 98(28). London: DoH.

Department of Health (1998e) *Smoking Kills*. White Paper. London: Stationery Office.

Department of Health (1998f) *Modernising Health and Social Services*. London: Stationery Office.

Department of Health (1999a) *Children Looked After by Local Authorities. Year ending 31 March, 1998, England*. London: Government Statistical Services.

Department of Health (1999b) *Children and Young People on Child Protection Registers. Year ending 31 March, 1999, England*. London: Government Statistical Services.

Department of Health (1999c) *The Government's Objectives for Children's Social Services*. London: Stationery Office.

Department of Health (2000) *Quality Protects*. Issue 4 (April): 9.

Department of Health/Home Office/Department for Education and Employment (1999) *Working Together To Safeguard Children*. London: Stationery Office.

Department of Health/Department for Education and Employment/Home Office (2000) *Framework for the Assessment of Children in Need and their Families*. London: Stationery Office.

Department of Social Security (1999) *Opportunity for All. Tackling Poverty and Social Exclusion.* London: Stationery Office.

Drakeford, M. (2000) *Privatisation and Social Policy.* Harlow: Longman/Pearson Education.

Dutt, R. (2000) Assertive, but sensitive. *Community Care,* (18–24 May): 32.

Evers, H., Cameron, E. and Badger, F. (1994) Inter-professional work with old and disabled people. In Leathard, A. (ed.) *Going Inter-Professional.* London: Routledge.

Fuller, R. (1992) *In Search of Prevention.* Aldershot: Avebury.

Hardiker, P., Exton, K. and Barker, M. (1991) *Policies and Practice in Preventive Child Care.* Aldershot: Avebury.

Hardiker, P., Exton, K. and Barker, M. (1999) Children still in need, indeed: prevention across five decades. In Stevenson, O. (ed.) *Child Welfare in the UK.* Oxford, Blackwell Scientific.

Hoyes, L., Lart, R., Means, R. and Taylor, M. (1994) *Community Care in Transition.* London: Community Care/Joseph Rowntree Foundation.

Hudson, B. (2000) Inter-agency collaboration: a sceptical view. In Brechin, A., Brown, H. and Eby, M.A. (eds) *Critical Practice in Health and Social Care.* London: Sage.

Macdonald, G. (2000) *What Works in Child Protection?* Essex: Barnardo's.

Parker, R.A. (ed.) (1980) *Caring for Separated Children.* London: Macmillan.

Siddall, R. (1994) Fag end. *Community Care,* (24 February): 16–17.

Social Exclusion Unit (1999) *Teenage Pregnancy.* London: Stationery Office.

Stone, K. (1994) The 'at risk' trap. *Community Care,* (10–16 November): 16–17.

Thompson, A. (2000) Falling through the gap. *Community Care,* (30 March–5 April): 20–1.

Tinker, A. (1990) Planning for a new generation of older people. In Carter, P. et al. (eds) *Social Work and Social Welfare.* Buckingham: Open University Press.

Tudor, K. (1996) *Mental Health Promotion.* London: Routledge.

Valios, N. (1999) Pointing the way to independent living. *Community Care,* (27 April–3 May): 24–5.

Wilson, M. and Francis, J. (1997) *Raised Voices: African-Caribbean and African Users' Views and Experiences of Mental Health Services in England and Wales.* London: MIND.

World Health Organization (1986) *The Ottawa Charter.* Ottawa: WHO.

World Health Organization (1998) *Health 21. The Health for All Policy for the WHO European Region.* Geneva: WHO.

CHAPTER 10

Promoting Physical Activity with Local Authorities

ROBIN IRELAND

The past 10 years have seen a tremendous surge in interest in promoting physical activity, influenced to some extent by the findings of health surveys, for example the *Allied Dunbar National Fitness Survey*, published in 1992, which showed that the majority of the English adult population took insufficient exercise for their health (Sports Council/HEA, 1992).

A Health Education Authority (HEA) symposium in 1994 made recommendations to individuals on appropriate levels of physical activity:

> Take 30 minutes of moderate intensity physical activity ... on at least five days of the week. (Killoran et al., 1994: xiv)

In 1996, the US Surgeon General reinforced the message that even a low level of physical activity achieves some benefit. At policy level, physical activity was granted more prominent status:

> Physical activity ... joins the front ranks of essential health objectives, such as sound nutrition, the use of seat belts, and the prevention of adverse health effects of tobacco. (US Department of Health and Human Services, 1996: v)

Since 1996, the emphasis has moved firmly away from sport towards encouraging physical activity as part of our daily lifestyle. Local authorities are key agencies in assisting the development of the physical environment in order to help the population to become more active. In addition, health at work policies have helped organisations consider the needs of their staff. Meanwhile the proliferation of government papers and programmes to address inequality and social exclusion has enabled new funding sources to promote physical activity. In primary healthcare, general practitioner (GP) exercise referral schemes multiply across the country.

Promoting physical activity in government

Department of Health

Increasing inactivity produces a range of health problems, including obesity and a higher risk of coronary heart disease and hypertension.

Saving Lives: Our Healthier Nation (DoH, 1999) considered physical activity from the disease perspective of coronary heart disease and stroke. The White Paper used the *Allied Dunbar National Fitness Survey* (Sports Council/HEA, 1992) data to report that 6 out of 10 men and 7 out of 10 women are not physically active enough to benefit their health.

The *National Service Framework for Coronary Heart Disease* provides a framework for tackling heart disease. Its Standard 1 says that:

> The NHS and partner agencies should develop, implement and monitor policies that reduce the prevalence of coronary risk factors in the population, and reduce inequalities in risks of developing heart disease. (DoH, 2000: 17)

Local authorities are recognised as key partner agencies. Framework interventions include encouraging public agencies to provide healthy workplaces that will provide staff with opportunities for physical activity. Service models include the production of local Health Improvement Programmes. An immediate priority for implementation is that by April 2001 all National Health Service (NHS) bodies, working closely with local authorities, will have agreed to and be contributing to an increasing physical activity policy.

Department for Culture, Media and Sport

It has never been clear exactly where sport fits at national level, having jumped between government departments in previous years. In its current home, sport is very clearly about success in competition and the winning of medals internationally. With this objective in mind, *A Sporting Future for All* (DCMS, 2000) is not about promoting physical activity for its health benefits. There is a shared objective, however, in that, to achieve excellence, it is understood that the participation base must be widened.

Sport also recognises that health provides an essential bargaining tool in winning support for local authority leisure development, from cardiovascular-based health and fitness suites to new swimming pools. Thus, while the new Manchester pool for the 2002 Commonwealth Games, in Oxford Road, and Ponds Forge, Sheffield, built for the World Student Games, have Olympic-standard facilities, they also have community facilities to meet the needs of their local population.

Sport England (1999: 3), with the support of the Local Government Association, argued that 'sport... can prove to be one of the "best buys" in preventive and rehabilitative health care'.

Department for the Environment, Transport and the Regions

Green transport is a key issue in the first decade of the new millennium. British roads are choked with cars, and while our children are increasingly inactive, 20 per cent of traffic can be traced to adults making the 'school run' (cited in Davis, 1999). The government's White Paper on the future of transport, *A New Deal for Transport: Better for Everyone* (DETR, 1998), made direct links between physical activity and transport, stating clearly that the way we travel is making us a less healthy nation.

New local transport plans are an essential part of the government's approach. On Merseyside, a partnership of five district authorities (the City of Liverpool, Knowsley, Sefton, St Helens and Wirral MBC) was engaged in 2000 in developing an integrated 10-year strategy that included a 'road user hierarchy', pedestrians and cyclists taking priority. There is a stated intention to develop Merseyside Walking and Cycling Strategies (Merseyside Connections, 2000). *The National Cycling Strategy* was produced in 1996 (DoT, 1996) and *The National Walking Strategy* in 2000 (DETR, 2000).

Other government opportunities

It is worth noting that there have also been developments in physical activity at European level. The European Union Health Monitoring Programme is developing physical activity initiatives such as European Physical Activity Surveillance Systems to assess information on national physical activity participation. The World Health Organization's Healthy Cities programme has also helped to develop local public health strategies.

At regional level in England, regional assemblies have a role to play. Health Task Group North West (1999) produced *Health: A Regional Development Agenda*, which considers a regional agenda for health. It identifies the important role that transport has to play in promoting health, including encouraging cycling and walking.

Promoting physical activity in local alliances

The government's clear lead through its three departments identified above has assisted local developments in health, sport and transport, in which local authorities have key roles to play.

Promoting physical activity through primary healthcare

Local authority leisure centres frequently offer a referral point for primary healthcare workers who wish to give their patients an exercise prescription. The link between diagnostic medical services and leisure provision can be traced back to the Peckham Health Centre in the 1920s and 30s (Scott-Samuel, 1990). This pioneering health centre had consulting rooms, a gymnasium and a swimming pool within the same building. Subsequent projects, such as the Health and Recreation Team in Liverpool (Sports Council, 1987), took referrals from health workers and gave patients a series of exercise options.

Primary healthcare workers hold a unique position in identifying and influencing those patients who may best benefit from increased physical activity. A report commissioned by the HEA (Biddle et al., 1994) found at least 121 primary healthcare schemes promoting physical activity in England. Their research also shows, however, that the schemes only reach a very small proportion of the patient base. Care must be taken in setting up protocols for such schemes so that GPs, Primary Care Groups and leisure services staff are clear about their objectives. GPs may, for example, refer patients who have multiple risk factors (hypertension and obesity for instance) for coronary heart disease, while leisure centre managers may simply have fastened onto an idea that they hope will help to fill their off-peak time.

Riddoch et al. (1998: 4) reached many of the same conclusions but also reported that schemes are often perceived as being very successful:

> Patients find support, a social life, and self-confidence. Patients experience an improved quality of life. Patients suffering from anxiety or depression are seen to benefit particularly. Individualised prescriptions and supervision are seen as important factors, particularly for patients who are initially fearful of exercise.

There has been concern expressed that leisure centres are not necessarily the best setting for activity promotion (Riddoch et al., 1998). The British Heart Foundation and the Countryside Agency have developed a Walking the Way to Health initiative, sometimes led by local GP surgeries and health centres. British Trust for Conservation Volunteers (BTCV) have designed Green Gyms (Trchalik, 1999) as an alternative to referrals to gyms and sports centres. They offer people 'the opportunity to improve their physical fitness by involvement in practical conservation activities such as planting hedges, creating wildlife gardens or improving footpaths' (Trchalik, 1999: back cover). A further option is the development of GP exercise referral schemes in Healthy Living Centres, another government initiative.

Local authority leisure centres are, however, likely to remain the most popular option for primary care schemes. For these to be successful, Riddoch et al. conclude that appropriate training is essential for both primary care and referral staff.

Promoting physical activity through sports development

Sports development officers are engaged in promoting access to sporting opportunities for all sections of the community. They are most commonly employed by local authorities but may also be employed by a governing body of sport. In 2000, The National Association for Sports Development was formed to provide support, advocacy and professional development for those involved in the development of sport. In North West England, a North West Health and Physical Activity Officers Forum has been set up with the objective of bringing together local authority officers engaged in promoting physical activity.

As has been recognised in many Sports Council reports, participation in sport is influenced by gender, race and disability, as well as by socio-economic status. Sport England (1999: 7) reports that:

> In Britain in 1996 those in the professional socio-economic group were almost three times as likely to participate in sport (excluding walking) as those in the unskilled manual socio-economic group.

Coggins et al. (1999) have addressed physical activity and inequality issues. A targeted approach may be adopted by sports development officers, among others, in order to engage specific members of the community in, for example, women-only swimming sessions, or popular Asian sports such as kabaddi. These authors suggest that:

> Exercise referral scheme coordinators who aim to reach isolated older people may need to consider transport to and from exercise facilities in addition to the normal activities necessary to encourage sedentary individuals to be more active. (p. 12)

Beishon and Nazroo (1997) report that Pakistani and Bangladeshi women suggested the existence of women-only facilities to be an important factor in influencing their exercise. Women-only facilities were also popular with both Indian and African-Asian women.

The Greenbank Sports Academy in Merseyside has shown how facilities can be designed, staffed and used by the whole community, including those with physical impairments and learning disabilities.

As noted earlier, it has been stated in the *National Service Framework for Coronary Heart Disease* (DoH, 2000) that, by April 2001, all NHS bodies, working closely with local authorities, will have agreed to and be contributing to an increasing physical activity policy. Some districts have already established physical activity strategies reflecting partnerships 'between the local authority, health services, voluntary sector and business community' (Wigan Council, 2000: 2). Wigan's strategy adopts a settings approach to promote physical activity, working in neighbourhoods, schools and workplaces.

Sefton Leisure Services and Sefton Health Authority have also formed a healthy alliance and produced an Exercise and Health Project Strategy (Sefton Leisure Services, 1998). Their programme has included providing effective exercise opportunities for children aged 7–12 years (Sefton Leisure Services, 1999), a particularly important target group given increasing evidence of obesity among school-aged children. Health Links, Wirral's Specialist Health Promotion Service, has developed physical activity initiatives including a successful Exercise on Prescription scheme. The service is jointly commissioned by Wirral Health Authority and the Metropolitan Borough of Wirral.

Events and promotional campaigns may be used to enable physical activity messages to reach the wider population. The Active for Life programme in England was effective in the late 1990s in promoting the message of moderate exercise to achieve health gain to health professionals. At a regional level, Healthstart's promotional events in the North West enabled it to gain an NHS Beacon Award in Health Improvement in 1999. Events such as the Liverpool Cycle Show, commissioned by Liverpool City Council with the support of key agencies such as Merseytravel and local cycling groups, have enabled health promotion messages to be communicated to a wider audience (Ireland, 1999). Healthstart's successful lifestyle festivals have been developed in partnership with NHS organisations, local authorities and organisations such as the Oldham Chamber of Commerce.

Promoting physical activity through green transport

The increasing use of cars has led directly to a decline in physical activity, as well as increasing environmental health problems. Local authorities, in addition to some health organisations, are beginning to address green transport issues. There are many examples of good practice across the country involving transport planners and policy makers, Local Agenda 21 officers and environmental health officers, directors of public health, health policy managers and primary care managers.

A Greater Manchester Guide has been produced to assist companies to implement Green Transport Plans, which includes measures to promote walking and cycling (Association of Greater Manchester Authorities, 1999). At a national level, *Making T.H.E Links* (Hamer, 1999) aims to outline the links being made by national government policies and to provide a framework for action by local authorities and health authorities.

At an international level, Sallis et al. (1998) have reviewed environmental and policy interventions to promote physical activity. In Glasgow, simply placing signs encouraging stair use next to escalators had a measurable impact on encouraging physical activity behaviour change (Blamey et al., 1995).

Active Transport (Davis, 1999) describes a number of positive transport initiatives including an NHS project in Stockport to promote walking and cycling throughout the borough. A Project Officer is employed for 22 hours per week to promote walking and cycling as part of everyday living. The job involves close liaison with a broad range of professions, including local authority staff and community leaders.

Following the launch of the National Cycling Network in 2000, with 5000 miles of new routes in Britain being developed, the task is to persuade people to leave their cars at home and try cycling and walking. Promotional campaigns such as Travelwise, and national events such as Walking to School Weeks (Pedestrians Association, 2000), all assist local authorities and health organisations in making the case for green transport.

Effective physical activity interventions

As has been seen, local authorities are very actively involved in promoting physical activity in different ways. There is still little evidence to determine the most effective form of intervention, and this must generally be determined by local partnerships agreeing local objectives through a process of consultation.

Whether the intervention is through GP referral schemes, the development of sports development and physical activity strategies, or cycling and walking forums, it is important, wherever possible, to measure its impact.

References

Association of Greater Manchester Authorities (1999) *Green Transport Plans. A Greater Manchester Guide.* Manchester: AGMA.

Beishon, S. and Nazroo, J.Y. (1997) *Coronary Heart Disease: Contrasting the Health Beliefs and Behaviours of South Asian Communities.* London: HEA.

Biddle, S., Fox, K. and Edmunds, L. (1994) *Physical Activity Promotion in Primary Health Care in England: Final Research Project for Health Education Authority.* London: HEA.

Blamey, A., Mutrie, N. and Aitchison, T. (1995) Health promotion by encouraged use of stairs. *British Medical Journal,* **311**: 289–90.

Coggins, A., Swanston, D. and Crombie, H. (1999) *Physical Activity and Inequalities. A Briefing Paper.* London: HEA.

Davis, A. (1999) *Active Transport. A Guide to the Development of Local Initiatives to Promote Walking and Cycling.* London: HEA.

Department for Culture, Media and Sport (2000) *A Sporting Future for All.* London: DCMS.

Department for the Environment, Transport and the Regions (1998) *A New Deal for Transport: Better for Everyone.* The Government's White Paper on the Future of Transport. London: DETR.

Department for the Environment, Transport and the Regions (2000) *Encouraging Walking: Advice to Local Authorities.* London: DETR.

Department of Health (1999) *Saving Lives: Our Healthier Nation.* London: Stationery Office.

Department of Health (2000) *National Service Framework for Coronary Heart Disease.* London: Stationery Office.

Department of Transport (1996) *The National Cycling Strategy.* London: Stationery Office.

Hamer, L. (1999) *Making T.H.E Links. Integrating Sustainable Transport, Health and Environmental Policies: A Guide for Local Authorities and Health Authorities.* London: HEA.

Health Task Group North West (1999) *Health: A Regional Development Agenda. Report of the Health Task Group (North West).* Liverpool: Liverpool Health Authority.

Ireland, R. (1999) Healthy return. *Leisure Manager,* (September): 14–15.

Killoran, A.J., Fentem, P. and Caspersen, C. (eds) (1994) *Moving On. International Perspectives on Promoting Physical Activity.* London: HEA.

Merseyside Connections (2000) *Merseyside Local Transport Plan Consultation. Stage Two Key Issues Paper.* Liverpool: Merseytravel.

Pedestrians Association (2000) *Taking the Strategy Step. Preparing a Local Walking Strategy.* London: Pedestrians Association.

Riddoch, C., Puig-Ribera, A. and Cooper, A. (1998) *Effectiveness of Physical Activity Promotion Schemes in Primary Care: A Review.* London: HEA.

Sallis, J.F., Baumann, A. and Pratt, M. (1998) Environmental and policy interventions to promote physical activity. *American Journal of Preventive Medicine,* **15**(4): 379–97.

Scott-Samuel, A. (ed.) (1990) *Total Participation, Total Health: Reinventing the Peckham Health Centre for the 1990s.* Edinburgh: Scottish Academic Press.

Sefton Leisure Services Department/Sefton Health Authority (1998) *Exercise and Health Project Strategy Document 1998–2005.* Southport: Sefton Leisure Services Department.

Sefton Leisure Services Department/Sefton Health Authority (1999) *Kids Excel Evaluation Report.* Southport: Sefton Leisure Services Department.

Sport England (1999) *Best Value Through Sport. The Value of Sport to the Health of the Nation.* London: Sport England.

Sports Council, Health and Recreation Team (HART) (1987) *Mersey Regional Health Authority; Phase 2 Monitoring Report.* Manchester: Sports Council.

Sports Council/Health Education Authority (1992) *Allied Dunbar National Fitness Survey: Main Findings.* London: Sports Council/HEA.

Trchalik, Y. (1999) *A Practical Guide to Setting up a Green Gym.* Wallingford: BTCV.

US Department of Health and Human Services (1996) *Physical Activity and Health: A Report of the Surgeon General.* Atlanta, GA: US Department of Health and Human Services, Centers for Disease Control and Prevention.

Wigan Council/Wigan and Bolton Health Authority/Wigan and Leigh NHS Trust (2000) *A Physical Activity Strategy for the Borough of Wigan 2000–2005.* Wigan: Wigan Council.

PART IV

EDUCATION AND YOUTH ORGANISATIONS

INTRODUCED AND EDITED BY ANGELA SCRIVEN

The targeting of young people for health promotion is regarded as being fundamentally important. This section offers an assessment of why this is the case and proffers a detailed evaluation of the possibilities for and constraints on such work in the locations where professionals engage in health-promoting activities: schools, colleges, universities and youth work settings.

Three chapters centre on schools. Each has a different focal point, collectively providing a broad picture of the current state of health promotion in the school setting. The first of these chapters focuses on education policy and how this influences the extent and nature of health-promoting activity in the curriculum. The revised chapter from the first edition of the book written five years ago makes it apparent that the policy agendas are different. There was a sense of despondency in 1995, but the current impression is that there is more to be optimistic about and a greater indication of government commitment to personal, social and health education in the new national curriculum. This is not a shift into complacency. The chapter ends with a plea that more needs to be done, but the mood is generally positive and the views expressed reflect affirmative change.

Beattie's update of his original chapter on health-promoting schools offers an interesting insight into how the movement has grown and developed over the intervening years since the first edition of the book. With its focus on curriculum matters, this chapter complements the preceding one. Beattie offers a fascinating mix of theory linked to discussions on the implementation and evaluation of health-promoting schools. The application of some of the new conceptual frameworks for planning and evaluating health-promoting schools, as well as the new ways of partnership working that this initiative encourages, suggests exciting times ahead for those working with young people in schools.

These positive views are unfortunately not advanced in the chapter on the health-promoting role of the school nurse. Farrow hints in the concluding elements of his chapter, following his assessment of the impressive functions of the school nurse, that the school nursing service is in danger of disappearing. Given Beattie's call in the preceding chapter for new and creative

113

ways of working for health and education professionals, the loss of the school nursing service would most certainly have an impact on the overall capacity of schools to engage in holistic health promotion with young people.

The final two chapters in this section move beyond initiatives located in the statutory education sector, by offering in one an overview and evaluation of the health-promoting universities initiative, and in the other an assessment of the role of the youth work sector in promoting health. The informal nature of the encounters with young people that youth workers enjoy makes it a highly appropriate environment for health promotion. The value of this setting in addressing health promotion targets is evidenced in the numerous case studies of good practice presented by the author, Robertson.

The health-promoting university is a fairly new initiative. The fact that the government does not specifically mention the role of universities in health policy is made more surprising when one reads Thompson and Dooris' account of the effect of other, non-health, government policies on the unhealthy conditions in which university staff and students work. One is left with the impression that universities are in a unique position to provide a range of initiatives that have the potential to impact positively on the health of those who study and work within these complex organisations.

In summary, this section has much of interest for those who have a remit for health promotion with the youth population.

CHAPTER 11

The Influence of Government Policy on the Provision of Health Education in Schools

ANGELA SCRIVEN

The assessment in the first edition of this book of the impact of the existing government policy on the provision of health education in schools made for bleak reading (Scriven, 1996). Over a decade has now passed since the Conservative government, under Margaret Thatcher's leadership, proposed radical ideas for a major overhaul of the education system in England and Wales. These ideas were encapsulated into the Education Reform Act (ERA) (DES, 1987). The implementation of the ERA resulted in a major change to both the management of the education system and the curriculum of schools. More recent health and education strategies initiated by the current Labour government have modified the original Tory policies. This chapter revisits some of the issues addressed in the first edition while taking account of the new policy environment in making an overall assessment of the current position of health education in schools.

Professional consensus on health education

A professional consensus on the importance of health education in schools is well established. There is a long-standing agreement, for example, that schools are a key setting for the promotion of health (DoH, 1992, 1999; Denman, 1994; WHO, 1997; Moon et al., 1999; Rowling and Jeffreys, 2000; Sinkler and Toft, 2000). A number of reasons have been put forward in support of this claim. First, and in accordance with the preventative philosophy inherent in health promotion, it clearly makes more sense to encourage young people to adopt a healthy lifestyle than to attempt to change unhealthy behaviour patterns in adulthood (Alexander, 1994). The impetus for targeting young people's lifestyle is predicated on the suggestion that the risk factors for disease in adulthood often originate in early life (Hurrelmann

115

et al., 1995). Second, and more importantly, the school provides the ideal environment for delivering a properly planned and coordinated programme of personal, social and health education to young people on a large scale (Downie et al., 1990; Hagquist and Starrin, 1997).

Given these points, it is hardly surprising that a second area of general consensus concerning the health education curriculum in schools is that the years between the 1970s and 1990 proved to be a sustained period of growth and innovation. It is not the purpose of this chapter to provide a potted history of the development of the subject or, indeed, to make a case for the continued need for health education in schools; there are good examples of this elsewhere (see, for example, Tones and Tilford, 1990; Lewis, 1993; Emmett, 1994). Suffice it to say that, by the early 1980s, research carried out by Southampton University for the Health Education Council (HEC) on a 12.5 per cent sample of all state schools in England and Wales indicated that 91 per cent of the sample were either providing health education or intending to do so (Williams and Roberts, 1985). A later study undertaken by MORI and commissioned by the successors of the HEC, the Health Education Authority (HEA), found that 77 per cent of primary, 91 per cent of secondary and 94 per cent of special schools either had a health education policy or were planning to develop such a policy (MORI, 1989). It would appear, therefore, that by the late 1980s, at the time when the ERA was being implemented, the need for and commitment to health education was being demonstrated by its presence on the curriculum of most primary and secondary schools in the UK.

The effectiveness of this health education is not altogether clear. There is, however, evidence to suggest that there was during this time considerable innovation taking place. Tones (1988), for example, discussed at some length the gradual move away from the medical model, which dominated early health education programmes in schools, towards a greater emphasis on values and attitudes, and the importance of personal and social factors. This shift in focus and approach is demonstrated through the various programmes that became a feature of work in health education during this time. Leslie Button's (1984) *Developmental Group Work with Adolescents* and Hopson and Scally's (1981) *Lifeskills Teaching*, although initially designed for youth work settings and personal and social education programmes respectively, were fundamental in influencing the move towards a more experiential approach in health education and, as a consequence, in redefining the subject.

Why then after a period of rapid and inspired developments, did we observe during the 1990s a more pessimistic outlook on the future of health education in schools? The prevailing view, as depicted in professional and academic journals at the time, appeared to be that the immediate future for health education was uncertain (Lewis, 1993; Emmett, 1994; Scriven, 1995). There is little doubt that the shift in mood from one of optimism to one of despondency coincided with the implementation of the ERA. To understand why the Act resulted in a perceived negative impact on the delivery of the health education curriculum, one only had to consider the key elements of the reforms.

The National Curriculum and its impact on health education

The introduction of a National Curriculum was seen as the central thrust of the ERA. The 10 statutory core and foundation subjects, with their associated assessment, applied throughout the years of schooling in four key stages from the ages of 5 to 16. Health education was not designated as a statutory subject but was one of five cross-curricular themes intended to be taught through the foundation subjects and through separate provision (NCC, 1990). There was a criticism of the National Curriculum by those with a professional interest in health education because the subject was not singled out for separate provision (Tones, 1988; Whitehead, 1989). Generally, however, there was a good deal of support from teachers and professional bodies for the new developments.

Moreover, it initially looked as if health education might consequently have a strengthened position in the new curriculum framework. This was partly because the ERA required schools to provide a balanced and broadly based curriculum, one that not only raised educational standards, but also promoted the spiritual, moral, cultural, mental and physical development of children and prepared them for the opportunities, responsibilities and experiences of adult life (Assistant Masters and Mistresses Association, 1989). In addition and for the first time, health education had a small but nonetheless compulsory presence in the statutory orders for the science core subject, and schools were offered guidance on how to formulate health education policies and develop a coherent health education programme (NCC, 1990).

As the full impact of the curriculum changes became clear, however, support for the innovation by teachers and health educationalists dwindled. Early signs indicated that some teachers were buckling under the strain of implementing the changes (Coghlan, 1989), and this situation did not improve. Slater (1991) pointed to schools reeling from the demands of implementing the curriculum provision, of doing what Partington (1990) described as too much too quickly. Gillard (1992) blamed the situation on the absurdity of attainment targets and statements at 10 levels, constantly changing and presenting teachers with an enormous task of curriculum mapping and planning.

Perhaps more significantly, Gillard (1992) claimed that the National Curriculum had pushed teachers towards a more subject-orientated curriculum. It was this unfortunate emphasis on the appropriacy of subjects that undoubtedly led to what some saw as the marginalisation of health education. Mackenzie (1990) believed that statutory subjects were given priority by teachers because they had programmes of study that lead to a period of testing and close reporting at the end of each key stage. The statutory attainment tests linked to some of the subjects proved to be extremely time-consuming, further marginalising the non-statutory areas. A further criticism of the national assessment was that it encouraged the adoption of a formal classroom approach, as opposed to the informal, pupil-centred, teaching style that had become associated with the delivery of health education (Troyna and Carrington, 1990; Denman, 1994).

It was felt at the time, therefore, that health education, as a cross-curricular theme, had not been accorded the same status as the core and foundation subjects, with their statutory orders and assessment. As a consequence, health education would have no authentic or credible position in the curriculum. Furthermore, both Mackenzie (1990) and Ritchie (1990) argued that cross-curricular themes were too difficult to weave into an already voluminous subject fabric. This view was nevertheless not universally shared. Code (1990), for example, made a salient point when she described health education as being a subject that lent itself to being incorporated into other disciplines, and, in a similar way to Wragg (1990), illustrated her point by working through the science attainment targets.

For the most part, however, the dominant view appeared to be that the National Curriculum had constrained the position of health education. O'Conner (1991) pointed to one significant feature of this marginalisation: the concentration of resources on the delivery of the statutory areas, including resources for in-service training (INSET). Research funded by the HEA and undertaken by the National Foundation for Educational Research found that money for INSET courses was more likely to be available for the National Curriculum core and foundation subjects than for health education (HEA, 1993).

There were, therefore, perceived problems for health education in the National Curriculum even following the changes carried out as a consequence of the Dearing review (Brown, 1994; Dearing, 1994a, 1994b). These modifications were embedded into the Education Act of 1996, which superseded Part 1 of the ERA relating to the National Curriculum (Holt et al., 1997). A survey undertaken at this time had schools reporting difficulties in prioritising the development of health education (Denman et al., 1999). When the Labour government came to power, it charged the Qualifications and Curriculum Authority with reviewing the National Curriculum and advising the Secretary of State for Education about recommended change (QCA, 1999). At the time of writing, the proposals have been published (DfEE, 1999), and implementation began in September 2000.

In comparison to its predecessor, the revised National Curriculum has more to offer those with a commitment to and responsibility for health education. In the consultation document (DfEE, 1999), there are details of what the chairman of the Qualifications and Curriculum Authority refers to as important new areas of personal, social and health education and citizenship. Citizenship is destined to become part of the statutory orders from September 2002 and will as such provide a forum for promoting a greater understanding among pupils of the rights and responsibilities that underpin a democratic society. It will also play an important role in helping pupils to deal with difficult moral and social questions that arise in their lives. Government briefing on the introduction of citizenship sees it as being complementary to proposals for raising the status and effectiveness of personal, social and health education (Blunkett, 1999). When one reads the programmes of study for citizenship, it is easy to see the links to the promotion of health. When pupils develop skills relating to enquiry and communication, and of participation and responsible action, it is hoped that they will become more empowered individuals and more able to act as advocates for themselves and their families.

The National Curriculum handbooks also provide for the first time a national framework for the teaching of personal, social and health education (PSHE). These guidelines encourage schools to establish coherence, consistency, continuity and progression in pupils learning in PSHE, although once again the non-statutory nature might inhibit coherence, consistency and progression. Notwithstanding this, the guidelines offer a useful emphasis on skills and understanding, rather than simply knowledge, and appear to encourage the sort of life-skills approach that, as previously discussed, is now generally recognised as being more in keeping with health education.

Some features of the original National Curriculum have been maintained. The two broad aims remain the same, showing a continued relevance to health education of the second aim, with its emphasis on promoting pupils' spiritual, moral, social and cultural mental and physical development and preparing all pupils for the opportunities, responsibilities and experiences of life (DfEE, 1999). There is certainly an indication from these aims that the curriculum is designed to achieve what Hagquist and Starrin (1997) identify as the relationship between schools' more traditional duties of providing knowledge and education on the one hand, and their responsibility for health and social training on the other. Core and foundation subjects will continue to dominate, the statutory tests and associated league tables creating the complex difficulties that potentially result in the marginalisation of non-statutory subjects, as in the early stages of implementation of the ERA.

The science core statutory orders retain what looks like mainly topic-focused work on health, under Life Processes and Living Things (DfEE, 1999). Unfortunately, research suggests that this tradition knowledge-based approach has little effectiveness in terms of long-term health gain (see, for example, Klepp et al., 1994), holistic approaches being considered to be more likely to empower young people to make healthy choices and change their behaviour (Moon et al., 1999).

In addition to the National Curriculum subject constraints outlined above, a further impact of the ERA was the reduction of schools' powers in terms of curriculum planning and the increased involvement of the government and lay people in areas that were traditionally the domain of the teaching profession. This change in power and control resulted in an educational climate that some saw as being non-conducive to the enhancement of school-based health education (Denman, 1994).

This is particularly true of the sex education elements of PSHE. One example of the diminishing powers of teachers in relation to sex education was in evidence before the ERA. Section 46 of the 1986 Education Act gave school governing bodies the responsibility for sex education, other than the science statutory orders, and the right of veto in individual schools (DES, 1986). This empowering of lay people with regard to curriculum matters continued with Section 6 of the 1993 Education Act, which allows parents to request the withdrawal of their children from part or all of any lesson in which sex education is taught, with the exception of National Curriculum science (Morris et al., 1993). As with the 1986 Act, governors were charged with overseeing policy and keeping parents informed (Kingman, 1994; Green, 1998).

This is clearly not working as intended as a survey in Nottingham found that only 59 per cent of schools possessed written policies (Denham et al., 1999), and another recent survey in secondary schools in Bristol found that most sex education policies had serious defects (Pearson, 1999). In addition to the National Curriculum reforms, therefore, criticism has come from both educational and other professional groups of the government legislation in relation to the sexual health elements of health education (see, for example, *ASHEC News*, 1994; BMA, 1994).

Section 28 of the Local Government Act of 1988 is another area of policy dispute as it forbids local authorities from promoting homosexuality in schools and as a result inhibits the approach that teachers can take to sex education. A controversial plan by the current Labour government to repeal section 28 was recently defeated (Hartley-Brewer, 2000).

Changes in educational funding

In addition to the National Curriculum, the ERA contained substantial policy shifts in relation to educational funding. The move to both the local management of schools (LMS) and grant-maintained status (GMS) had implications for the provision of health education. The Act fundamentally challenged the role and function of the local education authorities (LEAs), delegating many of their powers to school governing bodies and putting central education support services at risk (Bash and Coulby, 1989). GMS schools were expected to buy in advisory services, and both GMS and LMS schools had control over their staffing and in-service budgets.

Given the vulnerability of health education as a non-foundation subject, research in the mid-1990s indicated that it was being marginalised in the setting of priorities in relation to staffing, in-service and advisory service needs (Jamison, 1993). The Labour government withdrew GMS status when they came to office, but LMS status with associated LEA funding constraints remains in place.

LEA health education advisers

Another outcome of the change in LEA function as a result of the ERA was evidenced in the results of a national research study monitoring the impact of the reforms. The findings suggested that LEA health education advisers felt compromised because they frequently had to generate income in order to justify their position post-ERA (Scriven, 1994). This situation appeared to be influenced by both the new funding arrangements set out in the ERA and the withdrawal of the government Grant for Education Support and Training (GEST) 12A/B, the specific funding originally given to combat the misuse of drugs, this support being provided through the LEAs by specially appointed health education coordinators. These coordinators worked closely with schools and, in many cases, also at the professional interface, establishing collaborative partnerships between schools, LEAs and other agencies.

In the early 1990s, following several years of GEST funding, considerable partnership initiatives were in place. It is hardly surprising therefore that when the government pronounced that it would terminate the grant, those with a vested interest in school-based health education considered it an outrage (Harvey, 1993; Lawrence, 1994). There were many curriculum and funding developments in the mid-to-late 1990s relating to drug education in schools which demonstrated that the initial concerns relating to these funding cuts were, to some extent, unwarranted. For further information on this, see, for example, Noble (1997) and the overview of British government policy on drug education by Allott et al. (1999), which cites an impressive range of government publications and strategies introduced during the 1990s.

Despite this, a direct outcome at the time of the government change to education funding was a dramatic reduction in the level of advisory support for health education (*Times Educational Supplement*, 1993). Given the points already made concerning the marginalisation of health education as a result of funding changes embedded in the ERA, this lack of freely provided advisory support compounded the problems. The funding changes also came at an inopportune time, the Department of Health calling for professionals from a range of settings to form healthy alliances to address the national targets set for health (DoH, 1992). There was evidence from a national audit undertaken in 1994 that the contradiction in policies between the different government departments was making partnerships between health (specifically health promotion specialists) and education more difficult to initiate and manage (Scriven, 1994).

The need for and recognised value of interagency collaboration still dominate national health promotion strategies and other initiatives (Bloxham, 1997; Brown, 1997; Joyce et al., 1997; DoH, 1999). There is currently what appears to be a political desire to change the way in which policy is developed and implemented in order to facilitate these collaborative partnerships. The 'third-way' rhetoric that dominates recent government strategies (see, for example, DoH, 1999) strongly promotes the partnership of individuals, communities and government. This is combined with aspirations for 'joined-up thinking', or seamless government (DoH, 1999), which ensures that government departments work more closely together, thus avoiding some of the contradictory policies that have in the past affected health education.

A good example of this in practice is the National Healthy Schools Standards that is being run jointly by the Department of Education and the Department of Health. This is an ambitious programme involving the 150 LEAs in England who will take forward a new set of standards, in partnership with their health authorities, with the aim of implementing an accredited healthy schools programme for all schools by March 2002 (*Healthlines*, 1999; Sinkler and Toft, 2000). This initiative could have a major impact on the future development of health education programmes in schools. It appears from the National Healthy School Standard Guidance (DfEE, 1999) that the standards implicitly incorporate an impressive range of health promotion principles similar to those outlined in Rowling and Jeffreys (2000) in their discussion of health-promoting schools. These include equity, consultation, collaboration, ownership and sustainability, as well as some newer concepts such as capacity building and social capital.

One criterion encompassing some of these principles will potentially have a significant impact on health education; this is that pupils' views should influence teaching and learning in PSHE and citizenship. Research undertaken by Aggleton et al. (1998) suggests that young people operate with an integrated concept of health and well-being that sets great store by social relations and social activity. Importantly, the findings indicate that a narrow focus solely on commonly defined priorities, such as the drug topics in the core science curriculum, may not meet the expressed needs of young people. This new government initiative therefore looks as if it will influence the health education work in schools in a very positive way, stimulating a holistic approach and creating exciting new partnership arrangements.

The initial training of teachers

Another area of government policy that appears to have influenced the delivery and development of health education in schools is the reform of initial teacher training (ITT) (DfE, 1993a). Two elements in particular have had a direct effect. The first is the move to a more school-based training. It is possible that the location of a significant element of training in schools could disadvantage training in health education if the subject is not prominent on the curriculum.

The second element is the criterion for accrediting ITT courses initiated by the Council for Accreditation of Education, which has marginalised health education in the curriculum for teacher training. As a subject, it is not allocated student numbers by the government, and, since the advent of the National Curriculum, both primary and secondary training courses have been measured against criteria that reflect the National Curriculum core and foundation subjects. The Williams and Roberts survey of health education in teacher education courses indicated that there was 'a great chasm in teacher education regarding the place of health education' (1985: 46); this situation does not appear to have improved. A more recent survey undertaken by Walsh and Tilford (1998) to explore the impact of the 1992 ITT reforms on health education provision in the training of teachers concluded that there was a diversity in the quality, duration and content of provision for health education in the professional training elements of these courses and that ITT staff perceived post-reform provision to be inadequate (Walsh and Tilford, 1998). There was, not surprisingly given the finding that the content and time allocation to health education in ITT courses had diminished, a perception that newly qualified teachers were less competent to deliver health education.

The recommendation from the Walsh and Tilford (1998) study was similar to that from Williams and Roberts' (1985) study a decade earlier – that there should be an explicit, compulsory national curriculum for health education in ITT. The Teacher Training Agency appeared not to have taken account of the Williams and Roberts findings when it established guidelines for initial teacher education programmes (DfE, 1993b). It will be interesting to monitor whether any future review of these guidelines will recognise the greater importance placed on PSHE and on the complementary citizenship statutory guidelines in the revised National Curriculum.

There is an obvious need to keep the research into the provision of health education in initial teacher education programmes up to date, as well as an equally important requirement to monitor the impact of the new revised National Curriculum on the extent and nature of health education in schools. Studies such as the survey of schools' sex education policies cited earlier in the chapter indicate that there is still much to be done, but there is more to be optimistic about than five years ago. There are well-established healthy schools award schemes that are believed to result in health gain for pupils (Moon et al., 1999). The new National Healthy School Standard outlined above offers exciting opportunities, coupled with the existing Health-promoting Schools initiative (see Chapter 12; Tudor-Smith et al., 1995; Thomas et al., 1998; Rasmussen and Rivett, 2000). When all of these are combined with the curriculum changes that have been the focus for much of this chapter, the position of health education in schools appears to be sound.

In conclusion, it is encouraging that recent changes in health and education policy appear to have secured a more dominant and appropriate place for health education in the curriculum of schools. Those professionals who have worked hard to defend and promote PSHE, including the policy makers with responsibility for education provision, have established a sound basis from which schools can embrace both a range of initiatives and the establishment of new priorities and partnerships, such as the National Healthy School Standards. From the preceeding analysis, it is clear that there is still much to do and numerous problems yet to be resolved, but the future for health education in schools in the early part of the 21st century nonetheless looks auspicious.

References

Aggleton, P., Whitty, G., Knight, A., Prayle, D. et al. (1998) Promoting young people's health: the health concerns and needs of young people. *Health Education*, **98**(6): 213–19.

Alexander, D. (1994) Adolescents and young adults: overview. *Preventative Medicine*, **23**: 653–4.

Allott, R., Paxton, R. and Leonard, R. (1999) Drug education: a review of British government policy and evidence on effectiveness. *Health Education Research*, **14**(4): 491–505.

ASHEC News (1994) January, Issue No. 1.

Assistant Masters and Mistresses Association (1989) The National Curriculum. 'The Education Reform Act'. *Focus: Guidelines for Teachers*, January.

Bash, L. and Coulby, D. (1989) *The Education Reform Act: Competition and Control*. London: Cassell.

Bloxham, S. (1997) The contribution of interagency collaboration to the promotion of young people's sexual health. *Health Education Research*, **12**(1): 91–101.

Blunkett, D. (1999) *Achieving Excellence Through the National Curriculum in QCA/DfEE: The Review of the National Curriculum in England; The Secretary of State's Proposals*. London: QCA.

British Medical Association (1994) Press statement 'BMA expresses concern that the new Education Act may undermine health of the nation' (25 February).

Brown, T. (1994) Talking the PSHE out of the National Curriculum. *Health Education*, November (5).

Brown, T. (1997) Opportunities for health and education to work together. *Health Education*, **97**(4): 146–8.

Button, L. (1984) *Developmental Group Work with Adolescents*. London: Hodder & Stoughton.

Code, T. (1990) Mapping health education topics in the NC. *Education and Health*, **8**: 71.

Coghlan, A. (1989) A bumpy path to the National Curriculum. *New Scientist*, **124**(1692): 23–4.

Dearing, R. (1994a) *The National Curriculum and its Assessment: Final Report*. London: SCAA.

Dearing, R. (1994b) cited in *News Focus*, *Health Education*, January, No. 9.

Denham, S., Pearson, J., Hopkins, D., Wallbanks, C. and Skuriat, V. (1999) The management and organisation of health promotion: a survey of school policies in Nottinghamshire. *Health Education Journal*, **58**: 165–76.

Denman, S. (1994) Do schools provide an opportunity for meeting the Health of the Nation Targets? *Journal of Public Health Medicine*, **16**(2): 219–24.

Department for Education (1993a) *The Government's Proposals for the Reforms of Initial Teacher Training.* London: DfE.

Department for Education (1993b) *The Initial Training of Primary School Teachers: New Criteria for Courses.* Circular number 14/93. London: DfE.

Department for Education and Employment (1999) *National Healthy School Standard Guidance.* London: DfEE.

Department for Education and Employment/Qualifications and Curriculum Authority (1999) *The National Curriculum: Handbook for Secondary Teachers in England.* London: DfEE/QCA.

Department for Education and Science (1987) *Education Reform Act.* London: HMSO.

Department of Health (1992) *The Health of the Nation – a Strategy for Health in England.* London: HMSO.

Department of Health (1999) *Saving Lives: Our Healthier Nation.* London: HMSO.

Downie, R.S., Fyfe, C. and Tannahill, A. (1990) *Health Promotion: Models and Values.* Oxford: Oxford University Press.

Emmett, V.E. (1994) The Future of Health Education. *Health Education,* (May): 13–17.

Gillard, D. (1992) Educational philosophy: does it exist in the 1990s? *Forum,* **34**(4).

Green, J. (1998) School sex education and education policy in England and Wales: the relationship examined. *Health Education Research,* **13**(1): 67–72.

Hagquist, K. and Starrin, B. (1997) Health education in schools – from information to empowerment models. *Health Promotion International,* **12**(3): 225–32.

Hartley-Brewer, J. (2000) Political correspondent column. *Guardian,* Tuesday 25 July: 1.

Harvey, J. (1993) Health and education: partners no longer? *Public Health Alliance News,* (Nov–Dec).

Health Education Authority (1993) *A Survey of Health Education Policies in Schools.* London: HEA.

Healthlines (1999) Schools get health standard. (Nov–Dec): 5.

Holt, G., Boyd, S., Dickson, B., Hayes, H. and Le Metais, J. (1997) *Education in England and Wales: A Guide to the System.* Berkshire: NFER.

Hopson, B. and Scally, M. (1981) *Lifeskills Teaching.* London: McGraw-Hill.

Hurrelmann, K., Leppin, A. and Nordlohne, E. (1995) Promoting health in schools: the German example. *Health Promotion International,* **10**: 121–31.

Jamison, J. (1993) Health education in schools: a survey of policy and implementation. *Health Education Journal,* **52**(2).

Joyce, R., Toft, M. and Winstone, E. (1997) Promoting health in secondary schools. *Health Education,* **97**(1): 9–15.

Klepp, K.I., Oygard, L., Tell Grethe, S and Veellar Odd, D. (1994) Twelve year follow up of a school based health education programme. *European Journal of Public Health,* **4**: 195–200.

Kingman, S. (1994) The new law on sex education. *Health Education,* (September): 4.

Lawrence, N. (1994) *ASHEC News,* (Jan) (1).

Lewis, D.F. (1993) Oh for those halcyon days! A review of the development of school health education over 50 years. *Health Education Journal,* **52**(3): 161–71.

Mackenzie, C. (1990) Cross curriculum dissentions. *Education,* **176**(18).

Moon, A.M., Mullee, M.A., Rogers, L. et al. (1999) Helping schools to become health-promoting environments: an evaluation of the Wessex Healthy Schools Award. *Health Promotion International,* **14**(2): 111–22.

MORI (1989) *Health Education in Schools*. Report to the Health Education Research Department, Public Health Division. London: MORI.

Morris, R., Reid, E. and Fowler, J. (1993) *Education Act '93: A Critical Guide*. London: AMMA.

National Curriculum Council (1990) *Curriculum Guidance 5: Health Education*. London: NCC.

Noble, C. (1997) Daring to drop D.A.R.E. *Health Education*, 97(5): 187–92.

O'Conner, L. (1991) Healthy nation: feeling the squeeze. *Education and Health*, 9(2).

Partington, J. (1990) Week by week. *Education*, 176(6 July).

Pearson, D (1999) Sex education policies in schools: the first hurdle. *Health Education*, 99(3): 11.

Qualifications and Curriculum Authority (1999) *The Review of the National Curriculum in England: The Secretary of State's Proposals*. London: QCA.

Rasmussen, V.B. and Rivett, D. (2000) The European network of health promoting schools – an alliance of health, and education and democracy. *Health Education*, 100(2): 61–7.

Ritchie, H. (1990) Out of the frying pan, into the teapot. *Education*, 176(23 November).

Rowling, L. and Jeffreys, V. (2000) Challenges in the development and monitoring of health promoting schools. *Health Education*, 100(3): 117–23.

Scriven, A. (1994) Results of a national audit of healthy alliances between NHS specialist health promotion units and schools/LEAs. Unpublished research report, Bath College of Higher Education.

Scriven, A. (1995) Not a good year for health education. *Health Education*, (January) (1): 28–32.

Scriven, A. (1996) The impact of recent government policy on the provision of health education in schools. In Scriven, A. and Orme, J. (eds) *Health Promotion: Professional Perspectives*. Basingstoke: Macmillan.

Sinkler, P. and Toft, M. (2000) Raising the national school standard (NHSS) together. *Health Education*, 100(2): 6–7.

Slater, D. (1991) Prospecting fools gold: auditing the curriculum. *Forum*, 33(2).

Times Educational Supplement (1993) January 8, as reported in J. Jamison (1993) Health education in schools: a survey of policy and implementation. *Health Education Journal*, 52(2).

Tones, K. (1988) The role of the school in health promotion: the primacy of personal and social education. *Westminster Studies in Education*, 11.

Tones, K. and Tilford, S. (1990) *Health Education: Effectiveness and Efficiency*. London: Chapman & Hall.

Troyna, B. and Carrington, B. (1990) *Education, Racism and Reform*. London: Routledge.

Tudor-Smith, C., Roberts, C., Parry-Langdon, N. and Bowker, S. (1995) A survey of health promotion in Welsh secondary schools. *Health Education*, 97(6): 225–32.

Walsh, S. and Tilford, S. (1998) Health education in initial teacher training at secondary phase in England and Wales: current provision and the impact of the 1992 government reforms. *Health Education Journal*, 57: 360–73.

Whitehead, M. (1989) *Swimming Upstream: Trends and Prospects in Education for Health*. London: King's Fund Institute.

Williams, T. and Roberts, J. (1985) *Health Education in Schools and Teacher Education Institutions.* London: HEC.

Wragg, T. (1990) You can do health education in the NC. *Education and Health,* **8**(Mar–Apr).

World Health Organization (1997) *Promoting Health through Schools: Report of a WHO Expert Committee on Comprehensive School Health Education.* Geneva: WHO.

CHAPTER 12

Health-promoting Schools as Learning Organisations

ALAN BEATTIE

The concept of the health-promoting school concerns not just the teaching on health matters that happens in classrooms, or the medical and nursing attention that pupils receive through school health services, but also the school as a total setting. A document that has been highly influential in professional thinking on this topic offered the following summary:

> The health-promoting school aims at achieving healthy lifestyles for the total school population by developing supportive environments conducive to the promotion of health. It offers opportunities for, and requires commitments to, the provision of a safe and health-enhancing social and physical environment. (WHO, 1993: 3)

The idea that the school as a whole institution is a suitable arena for action to promote health is not in itself new: it has a long history. From around 1900, schools in Britain became test-beds in which children, 'easily seen, easily examined, easily described' (Armstrong, 1993a: 396) were subjected to analysis and intervention in the name of wider regimes of public health. For the first 50 years of the 20th century, medical advice was a dominant influence on the architecture and management of schools. Earlier (19th-century) school buildings, invariably designed on a 'central-hall plan' for ease of surveillance and discipline, were replaced wholesale by a new 'corridor, quadrangle and finger plan' designed to meet the 'sanitary ideal' (Lowe, 1973). It was believed that this new layout would provide healthier ventilation and lighting, and it continued to dominate school architecture until the late 1950s. Around the same time in the early 1900s, new systems were brought in for the medical inspection of children and for the provision of physical drills and school meals, all of which consolidated a new emphasis on the health and hygiene of school pupils (Armstrong, 1993b).

Textbooks for the training of teachers continued into the early 1960s to deal with school premises as an aspect of hygiene and health education (see, for example, Gamlin, 1959; Davies, 1962). From the late 1950s to the late 1980s, however, this focus on the school environment as an influence on health, and indeed the use of the term 'hygiene', slipped down the agenda as attention shifted to pupils' lifestyles and the psychosocial origins of risk-taking behaviour such as smoking, drinking, drug use, relationships and sexuality. The more recent renewed interest in the health-promoting school is an example of the re-establishment of an ecological view of health that has been one of the hallmarks of the 'new public health' and the settings-based approach (Ashton and Seymour, 1988; Baric, 1993). It reflects a concern to address simultaneously both the individual lifestyles of pupils and the corporate environment of the school – a working example of health promotion seeking to deploy multi-disciplinary perspectives drawing on psychological and sociological, as well as biomedical, understandings.

Guidelines for planning

In British schools in the late 1970s and early 1980s, there was a wave of new curriculum development projects for health education. This led to the earliest observations on the need to follow through what was learned in the classroom so that it became a matter of practice throughout the whole school environment and in the daily life of the school (Williams, 1985).

As with many other aspects of the new public health, however, it was in European policy-making bodies that the idea of the health-promoting school was decisively disseminated. The Council of Ministers of Education for the European Community issued a resolution encouraging authorities within member states to make arrangements to develop schools as a setting for health promotion (EC, 1989), the European Network of Health-promoting Schools (ENHPS) being set up as a joint research and development initiative of the World Health Organization (WHO) European Office, the Council of Europe and the Commission of the European Communities. The ENHPS now involves nearly 40 European countries, the socio-ecological ideal clearly informing the 10 aims set out for this initiative in 1993 (Table 12.1).

In the UK, detailed guidance on the healthy school had first been issued in Scotland (Young and Williams 1989; SHEG, 1990). In England, new guidelines on health education introduced in 1990 (at the same time as the new National Curriculum) included a section on the whole-school approach that drew attention to the subtle messages that pupils receive about health from the daily life of the school, as well as to other factors that may impinge on its effectiveness as a health promotion setting, for example the organisation and management structures of a school, its physical environment and its links with the local community (NCC, 1990). In 1991, the Department of Health (DoH), as part of the Health of the Nation strategy, endorsed the idea of setting up a pilot network of health-promoting schools (DoH, 1991). Then in 1993, the Health Education Authority (HEA) issued its own 12 criteria that schools were encouraged to work towards. These were similar to those of the WHO (1993) but offered some distinctive observations on the importance of linking schools to wider health and welfare services (Table 12.2).

Table 12.1   Aims of the European Network of Health-promoting Schools

1. Provide a health-promoting environment for working and learning through its buildings, play areas, catering facilities, safety measures and so on.

2. Promote individual, family and community responsibility for health.

3. Encourage healthy lifestyles and present a realistic and attractive range of health choices for schoolchildren and staff.

4. Enable all pupils to fulfil their physical, psychological and social potential and promote their self-esteem.

5. Set out clear aims for the promotion of health and safety for the whole school community (children and adults).

6. Foster good pupil–pupil and staff–pupil relationships and good links between the school, the home and the community.

7. Exploit the availability of community resources to support action for the promotion of health.

8. Plan a coherent health education curriculum with educational methods that actively engage pupils.

9. Equip pupils with the knowledge and skills they need both to make sound decisions about their personal health and to preserve and improve a safe and healthy physical environment.

10. Take a wide view of school health services as an educational resource that can help pupils become effective healthcare consumers.

Source: World Health Organization, 1993

Table 12.2   Criteria for a health-promoting school

1. The active promotion of the self-esteem of all pupils by demonstrating that everyone can make a contribution to the life of the school.

2. The development of good relationships between staff and pupils, as well as between pupils, in the daily life of the school.

3. The clarification for staff and pupils of the social aims of the school.

4. The provision of stimulating challenges for all pupils through a wide range of activities.

5. The use of every opportunity to enhance the physical environment of the school.

6. The development of good links between the school, the home and the community.

7. The development of good links between associated primary and secondary schools to plan a coherent health education curriculum.

8. The active promotion of the health and well-being of school staff.

9. The consideration of the role of staff exemplars in health-related issues.

10. The consideration of the complementary role of school meals (if provided) to the health education curriculum.

11. The employment of specialist services in the community for advice and support in health matters.

12. The development of the education potential of the school health services beyond routine screening towards active support for the health education curriculum.

Summarised from HEA, 1993

Table 12.3   Key areas for action to create a healthy school

---

1. *Curriculum.* The school should be working towards the National Curriculum Council Guidance No 5. Its policies and programmes should be coordinated, comprehensive and progressive, and be reflected in the School Development Plan.

2. *Environment.* The school should promote a stimulating, clean and safe environment.

3. *Policy.* This should reflect the school as a health-promoting environment which is part of the wider community.

4. *Hygiene.* The school should promote hygienic practices.

5. *Safety.* The school should promote a safe environment, including physical, personal and psychological safety.

6. *Exercise and activity.* The school should offer a wide range of physical activities that are accessible to all and in which working towards an active lifestyle becomes an important cultural practice within the school.

7. *Food.* Pupils should be educated and encouraged to make healthy food choices.

8. *Smoking.* The school should be working towards a smoke-free environment.

9. *Management.* There should be a holistic approach to the management of health-promoting issues in the school.

Source: Mancunian Community Health NHS Trust Health Promotion Service and Manchester City Council Inspection and Advisory Service 1994

Many statutory agencies subsequently devised their own more detailed, itemised schemes for guiding and encouraging local work on healthy school initiatives (for an example, see Table 12.3).

Progress in implementation

From the foregoing discussion, it is clear that the idea of the health-promoting school quickly proved attractive to planners at international, national and local levels. Progress in implementation at the school level was, however, at first slow, and the health-promoting school concept was in the early 1990s often greeted by practitioners with a mixture of enthusiasm and caution. This can be seen in three comments (quoted in Beattie, 1991a: 14) from senior professionals interviewed in 1991 in a study for the HEA on the feasibility of setting up a Healthy School award/support scheme:

> the school as a health-promoting environment is a really good idea. It's a basis for a holistic approach and helps you attack double standards across the whole school community. Staff would welcome it too. (Deputy Head of a high school in Wigan)

> A health-promoting school scheme is a good idea. The problem will be to find time to do it… We scarcely touch health as an aspect of the whole school environment. (Health education coordinator in a high school in London)

Focusing on the school as a health-promoting environment should be the abiding principle. An award scheme would be very good in encouraging this – as long as it didn't fall into the trap of favouring a medical model. (Senior health promotion adviser for schools in Manchester)

A survey of a representative sample of primary and secondary schools in England carried out in 1992 by the National Foundation for Educational Research (NFER) found that there was widespread support for the idea of health education as an important function of schools, together with a recognition of the value of a health-promoting school (Jamison, 1993). It also, however, found serious concern about a shortage of suitably trained staff and about the lack of time and money to secure essential training, especially faced with what was seen as the marginalisation of health education by the statutory requirements of National Curriculum subjects (as discussed in Chapter 11). A series of studies in Wales similarly highlighted early difficulty in achieving action on health-promoting schools (Nutbeam et al., 1987; Nutbeam, 1992; Smith et al., 1992, 1994). They found that, despite widespread agreement on the value of health promotion activity, whole-school policies with regard to smoking had been developed in only a minority of schools. Policies for healthy eating had been developed in even fewer schools, while a genuinely active involvement of parents in school health promotion policies was rare. These studies in Wales also found that opportunities for in-service training were seen as being inadequate to support the implementation of good practice in connection with the health-promoting school.

The late 1990s saw this picture begin to change. In 1995 as part of the ENHPS project, the HEA, together with its sister bodies in the other three UK countries, selected 48 schools as pilot sites across the UK (16 in England) for the implementation of three-year development plans, with support from the four national health promotion bodies (HEBS/HBW/HEA/HPANI, 1996). Progress in these schools was evaluated by the NFER, the final report (Jamison et al., 1998) identifying a range of gains for the pupils in the participating secondary schools: higher self-esteem, healthier eating patterns, less bullying and less smoking and drinking. It also noted, but only in some schools, a greater willingness to deal with staff health, particularly action on stress, and a greater involvement of parents and local community agencies. The conclusion was reached that the health-promoting school helps to foster the features known to be characteristic more generally of the 'effective school' (Reynolds et al., 1993; Stoll and Mortimore, 1995), suggesting that when a school invests in health as an area for development, this can facilitate the establishment of shared school aims and higher expectations of pupils, which leads in turn to broad academic and social benefits.

The same conclusion was reached in a report on another HEA project that examined what strategies and resources can be useful in arriving at a common approach towards embedding health promotion in the overall management of secondary schools. This report argued that healthy schools *are* effective schools, and that by recognising the importance of pupils' personal and social development, and investing in it, such schools raise pupils' self-esteem as well as academic performance (Toft et al., 1996). The findings from these two projects were eventually drawn upon to produce a guide for professional practitioners and advisers in education and health, offering advice on how to improve and develop a healthy school (HEA, 1999).

Another important development since the mid-1990s has been the proliferation of regional Healthy Schools schemes, which have been reported to be successful both in local studies, such as in Nottinghamshire (Denman, 1999) and Wessex (Moone, 1999), and in a national survey (Rogers, 1998). There has by now emerged, according to Rogers, a consensus among professionals working at local level, both in the education and health contexts, that the health-promoting school is indeed a valuable concept and that Healthy School Award schemes are an acceptable way of supporting implementation.

It was in fact clear from the early 1990s that the best basis for implementing health-promoting schools schemes would lie in creating and maintaining a local alliance between schools and health services (Beattie, 1991a, 1996; Turner, 1994). A new driver for action on these lines has now been established jointly by the Department for Education and Employment (DfEE) and the DoH (DfEE/DoH, 1999), in the shape of the National Healthy School Standard, hosted by the HEA (2000). In the policy document, *Saving Lives: Our Healthier Nation* (DoH, 1999), schools were identified as a key setting for action to improve health, the Standard providing a new framework for education and health agencies to work together locally to support Healthy Schools work. The DoH set up eight pilot sites around England in order to explore how to build on examples of best practice and reflect local priorities (Rivers et al., 1999), also introducing an accreditation process specifying criteria that local Healthy Schools partnerships can use to judge success in their own local programmes. The DoH's own baseline estimate in June 2000 was that 10 per cent of all schools were taking part in a local Healthy Schools partnership. Its target was that by the year 2002 all local education authorities would be involved in partnerships through the new standard, and all schools would have the opportunity to participate in a local Healthy Schools partnership.

Lessons from evaluation

The previous section cited a number of research studies that have reported attempts to evaluate the health-promoting school idea in action. The evaluation of health education/promotion projects has generally long been known to be a challenging undertaking (Gatherer et al., 1979), faced with competing definitions of basic concepts and with multiple criteria of success or worth (Tones and Tilford, 1994; Peberdy, 1997). The studies cited earlier all take some trouble to qualify their conclusions, typically acknowledging that what they have been able to report has been necessarily selective, by no means comprehensive, conducted over too short a timescale to be confident of tracking all the changes resulting from project implementation, and dealing with situations that are too complex and unsettled to allow the easy identification, let alone quantification, of all the relevant variables. Most of the studies have, to a varying degree, opted for pluralistic evaluation designs, seen as a means of addressing the distinctive contexts and processes of each school, identifying and accommodating new insights as they emerge, and generating data at multiple levels that can answer the diverse questions asked by different stakeholders (Beattie, 1995a; Crosswaite et al., 1996; Parsons et al., 1996; Tones, 1996; Springett, 1998).

A recent study has, however, moved forward the debate about the evaluation of health-promoting schools in a significant way. This review was commissioned by the Health Technology Assessment Programme within the NHS Research and Development Programme, reporting on a major systematic appraisal of the literature on health-promoting schools, which employed the explicit and methodical search procedures that are familiar in effectiveness reviews in the evidence-based medicine sphere (Lister-Sharp et al., 1999). Like most reviews of this sort, however, it started with the randomised control trial as its gold standard for evaluative inquiry, and it excluded from review all studies that did not use controlled comparison or before-and-after designs, or did not report explicit health-related outcomes. Using these criteria, the researchers found only 12 studies worthy of review, only three of these being full-scale health-promoting school projects (as opposed to applications of the approach to specific topics, such as cardiac health). Of these three, only two (both cited earlier in this chapter) were UK-based, the third coming from the USA. Despite this distinctly parsimonious sample, the review arrived at some clear and modestly positive conclusions about the effectiveness of health-promoting school (HPS) initiatives:

> carefully and skilfully executed interventions following the HPS approach have the potential to improve children and young people's health. Given the relatively low cost of these interventions and their potential for improving health, further experimentation should be encouraged...The HPS initiative is new, complex and developing, and implementation of all the components may take several years in any one school. Studies of programmes combining the 3 domains of curriculum, school ethos and environment showed that these were more likely to be effective than those which did not. (Lister-Sharp et al., 1999: 24, 113)

The review goes on, however, to identify some troublesome issues of theory and methodology that are raised by research and development related to health-promoting schools, issues that, it suggests, need further debate:

> Studies of this approach remain methodologically challenging, and too little attention has been given to the way in which the intervention and the evaluation impact on each

other. There is a need for more widespread understanding of the aims of health-promoting schools as well as further debate on the optimum way of evaluating such interventions... The process of randomisation [necessary to conduct a randomised control trial] is difficult to reconcile with readiness to change, which is likely to be important in achieving the active participation of schools... [Research agencies should] encourage and enable further debate on the value of including studies using observational and qualitative methodologies in reviews of effectiveness of health promotion interventions... [They should also] ensure that process evaluation which describes the way in which programmes have been implemented is undertaken and reported in all studies of health promotion in schools... [and] ensure, in publications of studies of school health promotion interventions, that the following are reported: the theoretical basis or assumptions underpinning the interventions; the content of the interventions; and the process of delivery. (Lister-Sharp et al., 1999: 24, 113, 115–16)

One further major independent review, which focuses on literature from Australia and the USA and on the specific case of primary schools, comes to a somewhat similar conclusion:

health gains for primary school students... will most likely occur if a well-designed program is implemented which links the curriculum with other health-promoting school actions, contains substantial professional development for teachers, and is underpinned by a theoretical model. (St Leger, 1999: 51)

This review emphasises that the health-promoting school approach is necessarily multi-faceted, and suggests that a high degree of commonality is now emerging between the structural frameworks devised for such work in different regions of the world, amounting to a new theoretical paradigm; moreover, when only one or two of the building blocks of the approach are employed, without any understanding and application of these comprehensive and integrative frameworks, the full benefits are not achieved.

These various evaluation studies taken together – both the first-hand studies of health-promoting schools in action drawn on earlier, and these two secondary reviews – point to some significant lessons that have so far been learnt (see Table 12.4).

Frameworks for future development

It is vital to act upon insights such as those set out in Table 12.4 if health-promoting schools are to deliver all of their potential benefits and if they are to be made sustainable. Perhaps not surprisingly, they echo the kinds of wider paradigm debate that have become familiar to health promotion professionals over recent years: the shift from health education to health promotion; promoting emotional as well as physical health; using socio-ecological and organisation development models rather than just individual-

Table 12.4   Lessons from the evaluation of
health-promoting school (HPS) initiatives

1. HPS projects must be about more than just health promotion 'based in' schools: they must be school-wide and strategic, focused on improving the school as a whole and as a resource for the community.

2. HPSs are most successful when their activities are undertaken simultaneously, in parallel with one another, in several different domains (curriculum, environment, ethos, parent and community involvement). It may be helpful for local projects to put more emphasis on the 'capacity building' that is entailed in connecting health promotion to other initiatives and other priorities in school improvement.

3. Not only is the curriculum element not enough on its own, but it must also in itself go beyond information giving and focus on health-related skills (for example assertiveness, coping and problem solving), values and cultural awareness.

4. Those developing and evaluating HPSs have not devoted as much attention to mental/emotional and social well-being as to physical health. Local projects need to give greater priority to debating and negotiating these other goals of HPSs (including stress, morale, coping and the school ethos), as well as strategies for achieving them.

5. HPSs have been quite successful in focusing on the health and lifestyles of pupils but need to widen their horizons to give a higher profile to staff (their professional development and their health) and to the school as a workplace, both as a physical environment and as a social organisation.

6. Planning and implementing HPSs has been most successful when there has been more involvement of pupils (peers), of parents and of external agencies in the local community. HPSs need to undertake such bottom-up partnership work to counter-balance the traditional top-down approach to planning and delivery.

7. Those involved with HPS projects need to acknowledge more fully the links between the healthy school and the effective school in order to address explicitly how far and in what ways pupils' learning can be improved when effort is invested in improving health, and to clarify what counts as evidence of 'effectiveness' in the HPS.

8. Those involved with HPS projects need to make clear the theoretical basis of their interventions, and report fully and critically the approach or model(s) they are employing. There also needs to be fuller and wider debate in and around HPS projects on what goals or outcomes the HPS is seeking, and how these relate to the theoretical model(s) used.

9. There needs to be a greater appreciation of schools as complex systems, and a readiness to adopt and adapt more sophisticated theoretical models that can connect together both health concerns and criteria and educational concerns and criteria.

10. There needs to be an increased monitoring and evaluation of HPSs. This needs to be built into projects, to be more rigorous and creative, to take account of continuing debate on goals, processes and outcomes, and to illuminate these and other issues of theory.

istic and/or biomedical models to promote health; and the case for bottom-up as well as top-down strategies for action on health (Sidell et al., 1997; Weare, 2000).

Health promotion practitioners employ a number of conceptual tools of thought to get this multiplex approach firmly in place on planning agendas (Jones and Naidoo, 1997; Beattie, 2000). Table 12.5 illustrates one such methodology as applied to a health-promoting school, showing different strategies (down the first column) that need to be deployed simultaneously, each of them unfolded across the domains of corporate life in the school (across the rows). A similar structural framework has been adapted as guide-

Table 12.5 A contract for multi-faceted, multi-level development in a health-promoting school

At what level will it happen? / What to do and why?	Curriculum: content and pedagogy	Ethos: staff/pupil relations; access to information and decisions	Environment: physical space, facilities, support services	Institution: structures and systems of decision making and communication
Give information and advice – to redirect the behaviour of individuals and reduce personal risks to health	Talks, videos, seminars on current health topics and priorities	Clear information and guidance on how health risks and infractions of codes will be dealt with	Space and resources for health promotion; exhibitions, displays, events	Clear and decisive house rules and codes on risks related to smoking, safety, HIV/AIDS, alcohol, bullying and stress
Offer personal guidance and counselling – to support life review and to strengthen individuals in order to encourage self-directed change	Individual support and pastoral care; discussion, role play, interactive work on peer pressure and social and life skills	Provision of opportunities and support for self-review and self-help; informal ways of dealing with stress, 'corridor rage' and similar incidents in the emotional life of the school	Facilities for self-help and group work	Systems to support staff and pupils who need to adapt to rules and codes
Invest in outreach and liaison and networking – to identify common ground, strengthen community links and facilitate joint action	Courses for parents; links to adult and community education; staff support; challenge social exclusion in work with outside local agencies and with voluntary self-help schemes	Set up local networks; increase community participation; improve communication: school–home and school–community; open meetings and events	Labelling, signposting, way-finding for all visitors; briefings on environmental awareness	Act as statutory enabler: create or maintain supportive networks and infrastructures. For parent involvement: community service and volunteer schemes; visitor schemes
Take regulatory administrative action – to improve the environment: physical, social and cultural	Assignments and projects that link to the school building and grounds, as well as to the locality	Give access to information and decisions about the school environment and its impact on the locality	Offer community use of school facilities; liaison over issues of school grounds, roads and car use and journeys to school; 'greening the school'	Lobby and campaign to transform local environments; laws, regulations, policies; standards, plans

Source: After Beattie, 1984, 1991b, 1993, 1995b, 1996, 1997, 1998; O'Donnell and Gray, 1993

lines for delivering the Health of the Nation targets (Simnett, 1993) and as contracts for health improvement when implementing *Our Healthier Nation* targets (DoH, 1999).

A grid such as this can be used to structure dialogue on the different sorts of aim, purpose, procedure, target and underlying value and belief that diverse stakeholders bring to a health-promoting school project, and/or to prompt those involved to figure out which aims, activities and values they can agree on and take forward (Ewles and Simnett, 1992; Turner, 1994). It can be useful in joint planning, performance review and audit within local health-promoting school alliances and within wider managerial systems, local and national inspections, award schemes and so on. It is a way of keeping the full picture of strategic choices clearly in view.

A health-promoting school's work arguably needs a second framework of thought to assist in reviewing and structuring not just the content of its agenda, but also the process of setting and delivering that agenda. The contested ideas and complex coalitions in these schemes (see Tables 12.4 and 12.5 above) represent exactly the kind of challenge for which whole-systems thinking has been developed in management studies. This emerged from an enquiry into what it takes for organisations to respond speedily and intelligently to fast-changing and complex environments, its best-known example being the concept of the learning organisation: 'an organisation that facilitates the learning of all its members and consciously transforms itself and its context' (Pedler et al., 1997: 3).

In health promotion in general, the dominant theoretical perspectives have tended to be versions of social learning theory focused on development and change in individuals, and this has been true also of health-promoting schools' work (Lister-Sharp, 1999; St Leger, 1999). But learning organisation theory offers a starkly different view that is concerned with understanding and changing the organisational structures and cultures that shape the capacity to learn of the enterprise as a whole. As such, the learning organisation approach can offer a direct way of tackling typical agendas in this area for future action (see Tables 12.4 and 12.5 above). This framework can help staff to: 'extend their capacity for multiple viewing of organisational phenomena... to tolerate and deal with conflict... to learn to model good organisational dialectic' (Argyris and Schön, 1978: 313).

The learning organisation approach has been most fully developed by Senge et al. (1990, 1994, 1999), and it is striking that much recent innovation in professional practice in public health (such as Health Improvement Programmes, Health Action Zones and Healthy Living Centres) has either been modelled directly on Senge's work or has at least been strongly influenced by whole-systems thinking. One source of influence lies in the work of the King's Fund 'urban health partnership', which has experimented on many fronts with working whole systems (Harries et al., 1998, Plamping et al., 1998, Pratt et al., 1999), for example through whole-systems learning events and in building the capacity for effective collaboration in local partnerships for health (Plamping et al., 2000). A clear understanding of the conceptual foundations and operational practicalities of the learning organisation approach, and a readiness to use it, could give health-promoting schools new common ground with public health agencies and make the future implementation of such schemes more secure and sustainable.

Figure 12.1 shows the five disciplines through which information can be structured and shared in an organisation in order to manage processes of strategic change, by orchestrating a continuous interplay between public and personal forms of knowledge, and between individual and collaborative reflection-and-action. An organisational learning cycle like this could guide health-promoting schools through the messy, but no doubt essential and unavoidable, processes of 'muddling through with a model' (Beattie, 1997, 1998).

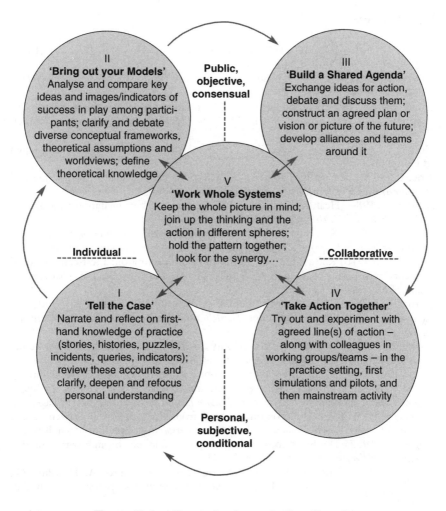

Figure 12.1 The cycle of organisational learning
(adapted from Boisot, 1994, 1995; Boisot et al., 1997;
Dixon, 1994; Senge, 1990, 1994, 1999)

The development of health-promoting schools appears to be making significant improvements to the health and well-being of children and young people and may also have important benefits for school staff, local families and communities. New conceptual frameworks for planning, implementing and evaluating health-promoting schools that are coming into use can make delivery more reliable and more sustainable. But these new developments will pitch health and education professionals into new ways of working, ways that are flexible, creative, cooperative and above all concerned with building the capacity for organisational change.

References

Argyris, C. and Schön, D. (1978) *Organizational Learning: a Theory of Action Perspective.* New York: Addison-Wesley.

Armstrong, D. (1993a) Public health spaces and the fabrication of identity. *Sociology,* 27(3): 393–410.

Armstrong, D. (1993b) From clinical gaze to regime of total health. In Beattie, A., Jones, L., Gott, M. and Sidell, M. (eds) *Health and Wellbeing: a Reader.* Basingstoke: Macmillan.

Ashton, J. and Seymour, H. (1988) *The New Public Health.* Buckingham: Open University Press.

Baric, L. (1993) The settings approach: implications for policy and strategy. *Journal of the Institute of Health Education,* 30(1): 17–24.

Beattie, A. (1984) Health education and the science teacher: invitation to a debate. *Education and Health,* (January): 9–15.

Beattie, A. (1991a) *Supporting School Health Education in the Context of the National Curriculum: A Research Report for the Young People's Programme.* London: HEA.

Beattie, A. (1991b) Knowledge and control in health promotion: a test-case for social theory and social policy. In Gabe, J., Calnan, M. and Bury, M. (eds) *Sociology of the Health Service.* London: Routledge.

Beattie, A. (1993) The changing boundaries of health. In Beattie, A., Gott, M., Jones, L. and Sidell, M. (eds) *Health and Wellbeing: a Reader.* London: Macmillan.

Beattie, A. (1995a) Evaluation in community development for health: an opportunity for dialogue. *Health Education Journal,* 54: 465–72.

Beattie, A. (1995b) The health promoting campus: a case study in project-based learning and competency profiling. In Edwards, A. and Knight, P. (eds) *Degrees of Competence: The Assessment of Competence in Higher Education.* London: Kogan Page.

Beattie, A. (1996) The health promoting school: from idea to action. In Scriven, A. and Orme, J. (eds) *Health Promotion: Professional Perspectives.* London: Macmillan.

Beattie, A. (1997) The health promoting campus: muddling through with a model. *Journal of Contemporary Health,* 6: 29–31.

Beattie, A. (1998) Action learning for health on campus. In Tsouros, A., Dowding, G., Thompson, J. and Dooris, M. (eds) *Health Promoting Universities.* Copenhagen: WHO.

Beattie, A. (2000) Health promotion. In Dowrick C. (ed.) *Medicine in Society: Behavioural Sciences for Medical Students.* London: Edward Arnold.

Boisot, M. (1994) *Information and Organization: The Manager as Anthropologist.* London: HarperCollins.

Boisot, M. (1995) *Information Space: a Framework for Learning in Organizations, Institutions and Culture.* London: Routledge.

Boisot, M., Griffiths, D. and Moles, V. (1997) The dilemma of competence: differentiation versus integration in the pursuit of learning. In Sanchez, R. and Heene, A. (eds) *Strategic Learning and Knowledge Management.* Chichester: John Wiley & Sons.

Crosswaite, C., Currie, C. and Young, I. (1996) The European network of health promoting schools: development and evaluation, Scotland. *Health Education Journal,* **55**: 450–6.

Davies, M.B. (1962) *Hygiene and Health Education for Training Colleges* (9th edn). London: Longmans.

Denman, S. (1999) Health promotion policies in Nottinghamshire schools. *Health Education Journal,* **58**(2): 215–19.

Department for Education and Employment/Department of Health (1999) *National Healthy School. Standard: Guidance Paper.* London: HMSO.

Department of Health (1991) *The Health of the Nation.* White Paper. London: HMSO.

Department of Health (1999) *Saving Lives: Our Healthier Nation* (Cm 4386). London: HMSO.

Dixon, N. (1994) *The Organizational Learning Cycle.* Maidenhead: McGraw-Hill.

European Commission (1989) Resolution of the Council of Ministers of Education, meeting within Council 23 November 1988, concerning health education in schools. *European Commission, Official Journal,* 9/c/3/01.

Ewles, L. and Simnett, I. (1992) *Promoting Health: A Practical Guide.* London: Scutari Press.

Gamlin, R. (1959) *Modern School Hygiene* (19th edn). Welwyn: Nisbet.

Gatherer, A., Parfitt, J. and Vessey, M. (1979) *Is Health Education Effective?* London: HEC.

Harries, J., Gordon, P., Plamping, D. and Fischer, M. (1998) *Elephant Problems and Fixes that Fail.* London: King's Fund.

Health Education Authority (1993) *The Concept of the Health Promoting School: The European Network of Health Promoting Schools – How your School can be Involved.* London: HEA.

Health Education Authority (1999) *Whole School – Healthy School: An Essential Guide to the Health Promoting School.* London: HEA.

Health Education Authority (2000) *Healthy Schools Programme* http://hea.org.uk/campaigns/hsp/hsmain.html

Health Education Board, Scotland/HBW/Health Education Authority/HPANI (1996) The European network of health promoting schools: introduction – the UK project. *Health Education Journal,* **55**: 447–9.

Jamison, J. (1993) Health education in schools: a survey of policy and implementation. *Health Education Journal,* **52**(2): 59–62.

Jamison, J., Ashby, P., Hamilton, K., Macdonald, A. and Saunders, L. (1998) *The Health Promoting School. Final Report of the ENHPS Evaluation Project in England.* London: HEA.

Jones, L. and Naidoo, J. (1997) Theories and models in health promotion. In Katz, J. and Peberdy, A. (eds) *Promoting Health: Knowledge and Practice.* London: Macmillan.

Lister-Sharp, D., Chapman, S., Stewart-Brown, S. and Sowden, A. (1999) Health promoting schools and health promotion in schools: two systematic reviews. *Health Technology Assessment*, **3**: 22.

Lowe, R.A. (1973) The medical profession and school design in England, 1902–14. *Pedagogica Historica*, **13**(2): 425–44.

Mancunian Community Health NHS Trust Health Promotion Service and Manchester City Council Inspection/Advisory Service (1994) *Manchester Healthy School Award Scheme*. Manchester.

Moone, A.M. (1999) Helping schools to become health-promoting environments: an evaluation of the Wessex Healthy Schools Award. *Health Promotion International*, **14**(2): 111–22.

National Curriculum Council (1990) *Curriculum Guidance 5: Health Education*. York: NCC.

Nutbeam, D. (1992) The health promoting school: closing the gap between theory and practice. *Health Promotion International*, 7(3): 151–3.

Nutbeam, D., Clarkson, J., Phillips, K., Everett, V., Hill, A. and Catford, J. (1987) The health promoting school: organisation and policy development in Welsh secondary schools. *Health Education Journal*, **46**(3): 109–15.

O'Donnell, T. and Gray, G. (1993) *The Health Promoting College*. London: HEA.

Parsons, C., Stears, D. and Thomas, C. (1996) The health promoting school in Europe: conceptualising and evaluating the change. *Health Education Journal*, **55**: 311–21.

Peberdy, A. (1997) Evaluating community action. In Jones, L. and Sidell, M. (eds) *The Challenge of Promoting Health: Exploration and Action*. London: Macmillan.

Pedler, M., Burgoyne, J. and Boydell, T. (1997) *The Learning Company: A Strategy for Sustainable Development* (2nd edn). London: McGraw-Hill.

Plamping, D., Gordon, P. and Pratt, J. (1998) *Action Zones and Large Numbers*. London: King's Fund.

Plamping, D., Gordon, P. and Pratt, J. (2000) Practical partnerships for health and local authorities. *British Medical Journal*, **320**: 1723–5.

Pratt, J., Gordon, P. and Plamping, D. (1999) *Working Whole Systems*. London: King's Fund.

Reynolds, D., Hopkins, D. and Stoll, L. (1993) Linking school effectiveness knowledge and school improvement practice: towards a synergy. *School Effectiveness and School Improvement*, **4**(1): 37–58.

Rivers, K., Aggleton, P., Chaise, E. et al. (1999) *Learning Lessons: A Report on Two Research Studies Informing the National Healthy Schools Standard*. London: DfEE/DoH.

Rogers, E. (1998) Developing the health promoting school: a national survey of healthy schools awards. *Journal of Public Health*, **112**: 37–40.

St Leger, L.H. (1999) The opportunities and effectiveness of the health promoting primary school in improving child health – a review of the claims and evidence. *Health Education Research*, **14**(1): 51–69.

Scottish Health Education Group (1990) *Promoting Good Health: Proposals for Action in Schools*. Edinburgh: SHEG.

Senge, P. et al. (1990) *The Fifth Discipline: the Art and Practice of the Learning Organization*. New York: Doubleday.

Senge, P. et al. (1994) *The Fifth Discipline Fieldbook: Strategies and Tools for Building a Learning Organization*. London: Nicholas Brealey.

Senge, P. et al. (1999) *The Dance of Change: The Challenges of Sustaining Momentum in Learning Organisations*. London: Nicholas Brealey.

Sidell, M., Jones, L., Katz, J. and Peberdy, A. (eds) (1997) *Debates and Dilemmas in Promoting Health*. London: Macmillan.

Simnett, I. (1993) *Delivering Health to the Nation*. London and Bristol: HEA/NHSTD.

Smith, C., Roberts, C., Nutbeam, D. and Macdonald, G. (1992) The health promoting school: progress and future challenges in Welsh secondary schools. *Health Promotion International*, 7: 171–9.

Smith, C., Frankland, J., Playle, R. and Moore, L. (1994) A survey of health promotion in Welsh primary schools 1993. *Health Education Journal*, **53**: 237–48.

Springett, J. (1998) Quality measures and evaluation of Healthy City policy initiatives. In Davies, J.K. and Macdonald, G. (eds) *Quality, Evidence and Effectiveness in Health Promotion*. London: Routledge.

Stoll, L. and Mortimore, P. (1995) *School Effectiveness and School Improvement*. Viewpoint No. 2. London: University of London Institute of Education.

Toft, M., Inman, S. and Whitty, G. (eds) (1996) *Healthy Schools Are Effective Schools: A Report on the HEA 'Promoting Health in Secondary Schools' Project*. London: HEA.

Tones, K. (1996) The health promoting school: some reflections on evaluation. *Health Education Research*, **11**(4): i-viii.

Tones, K. and Tilford, S. (1994) *Health Education: Effectiveness, Efficiency and Equity*. London: Chapman & Hall.

Turner, R. (1994) Purchasing practical health promotion for the primary school: a DHA perspective. In Morton, R. and Lloyd, J. (eds) *The Health Promoting Primary School*. London: Fulton.

Weare, K. (2000) *Promoting Mental, Emotional and Social Health: A Whole School Approach*. London: Routledge.

World Health Organization (1993) *The European Network of Health Promoting Schools: a Joint WHO/CE/CEC Project*. Copenhagen: WHO.

Williams, T. (1985) Health education and the school/community interface. In Campbell, G. (ed.) *New Directions in Health Education*. Brighton: Falmer Press.

Young, I. and Williams, T. (1989) *The Healthy School*. Edinburgh: SHEG.

CHAPTER 13

The Role of the School Nurse in Promoting Health

STEPHEN FARROW

When services become invisible, they run the risk of being reduced or even abandoned. During the 1980s and 90s, the school health service was such a service (Harrison and Gretton, 1986; While and Barriball, 1993), in many parts of the country suffering significant cuts. These changes came about partly because people believed that the improved socio-economic circumstances of children and families, when compared with their counterparts in the early decades of this century, did not require a service whose origins lay in poverty. They also resulted from a lack of clarity over the role of the school nurse and concern for the cost-effectiveness of the school health service.

The original role of the school nurse was to focus on the detection and treatment of poor hygiene, infestations and malnutrition, and to provide a supporting role to that of school medical officers. The 1944 Education Act had extended the work of the school nurse to the secondary school, the NHS Act 1977 confirming that the only statutory function with regard to schoolchildren was periodic inspection. The 1981 Education Act then integrated children with learning difficulties into ordinary schools and the National Curriculum (Thyer, 1996) introduced the requirement to provide for health education and health promotion. More recently, guidance on good practice in community child health services confirmed that the inspection of children could properly take place in primary care settings and was not required to be in school (DoH, 1996, 1997).

In general, the post-war period had seen increased opportunity and increased activity, particularly in the field of immunisation and health promotion. Concurrently, however, there was a reduction in the number of community medical officers working in schools and an alteration in the general relationships between nurses and doctors with the greater autonomy of school nurses. At the same time that opportunities have increased for school nurses to have a greater impact on the health of children, there has been a general questioning of their role and, more particularly, of the level of resources that should be allocated to children, schools, health education and health promotion.

There have nevertheless been some positive developments as a result of the Green Paper *Our Healthier Nation*, which emphasised the school as a key setting for improving the health of children (DoH, 1998). This approach is similar to that in New South Wales, Australia, where promoting better health in school is part of the National Health Strategy. In the UK, the health-promoting school is becoming an essential building block for the national health strategy (Thyer, 1996; see also Chapter 12). One aspect of the developing debate has been the training and education of school nurses themselves. Before 1974, most school nurses were trained health visitors, but the number holding this qualification has been steadily declining (Doggett et al., 1992).

Before describing the role of school nurses in health promotion and the current constraints on and opportunities for the development of their role, a brief review of the literature will be attempted. This begins with comments on the historical context and the organisation of school nursing services, as well as a discussion of the nurse's role. It is then followed by a brief reference to the debate concerning school medicals, school inspections and the screening interview. The next sections consider the general question of workload and training needs, and a series of specific issues that illustrate various expanding aspects of the current job. The final section deals with health promotion in particular and with what factors may influence its development. These differing roles and the variability in delivery at local level are emphasised in the findings of several authors (Bagnall and Dilloway, 1996a; Health Visitors' Association, 1996; DeBell and Everett, 1997).

Historical context and organisation

School nursing has been in transition since its inception, the role of the school nurse as primary care coordinator, school health coordinator, case manager and epidemiologist replacing outdated nursing functions (Igoe, 1994). In a contribution to the Whither health visiting series in *Health Visitor*, Bagnall (1989) concluded that the school nursing service needed a thorough review and update. Given the stated importance of the child at the political level and the emergence of key policy documents (Health Visitors' Association, 1988; Primary Healthcare Group, 1988), it was time for school nurses and managers to implement some of the changes that were obviously needed.

Another perspective comes from reports of school nursing services within different districts in England. In the mid-1990s, Norwich had one of the most comprehensive programmes of school nurse activity, including screening at entrance and systematically throughout the child's career, as well as health interviews. Discussions took place about future careers, special attention being given to medical conditions. There was an extensive programme of health education regarding diet, exercise, smoking and other relevant subjects. Counselling, if necessary, for any health, social and personal worries was also provided, as were drop-in clinics (Hawes, 1989).

Compared with Norwich, there were many districts with only a skeleton school health or school nursing service. It was also quite common to find two districts in the same region with a quite different approach to school nursing. In Bristol, in 1992, the policy was to reduce the number of school nurse establishments in order to buy in health promotion and to provide paramedical services for children with special needs. In contrast, in Exeter, the school nurse was placed at the heart of services for children (Jackson, 1992). A survey of National Health Service (NHS) Trusts providing school health services found that fewer than a third had developed a strategy for their school health service (Bagnall and Dilloway, 1996b).

In a number of districts, the school health service strategy involved the development of teams. In Stockport, the team consisted of health visitor, school nurse and healthcare assistant (Jackson, 1991); in Wandsworth, the team comprised a school nurse team leader, an additional nurse and a clerical officer (Turner, 1994); and in East Dorset, the team included a nursery nurse (Lochhead, 1994).

In the USA, both the history and the changes have been similar to those seen in the UK (Thompson, 1989; Barnfather, 1991; Thurber et al., 1991; National Association of State School Nurse Consultants, 1993; Brother, 1998; Gaffrey and Bergren, 1998; Hacker and Wessel, 1998; Klahn et al., 1998; Juhn et al., 1999).

Role of school nurses

Surveys of the views of pupils and staff on the role of the school nurse have shown that they tend to view the nurse in a traditional way, that is, caring for the sick and injured, whereas the nurses themselves tended to give priority to health surveillance, screening and the prevention of illness, together with health promotion (Staunton, 1983; Hansen, 1987, Adams, 1990). The views of parents differed in that they saw routine medicals, hygiene inspections and regular vision and hearing tests as being important (Adams, 1990). From these findings and those from North America, it could be said that parents had the most limited perception of the school nurse's role (Greenhill, 1979). Parents and teachers are often seen as authority figures, whereas the school nurse is viewed as an independent health professional. Cohen (1994) gives examples of collaboration between school nurses and teachers. A survey was conducted in Ottawa schools before the introduction of a compulsory AIDS education programme. Girls considered parents, and boys considered school nurses, to be the next most credible source of information (Dolan et al., 1990).

An important aspect of the role of school nurses is the extent to which they take a leadership role within the school. With the introduction of new programmes, such as the care of the pregnant teenager and substance abuse education, the school nurse became increasingly involved with other profes-sionals both inside and outside the school system. The nurses' effectiveness depended greatly on their ability to lead (Adams, 1991).

Despite the widening of the role, school nurse functions may not be that visible to schoolchildren themselves. A review of children in Bath showed that pupils entering secondary school were aware of who the school nurse was and how to contact her but were unaware of what she did (Williamson, 1992). Several authors have stressed the enormous variation in the role of the school nurse across the country and the competencies needed to make the role successful (Parsons and Felton, 1992; Yates, 1992; While and Barriball, 1993).

The Health Visitors Association's policy document *Project Health* was launched in 1991 to coincide with the first national school nursing week. It was the intention of the professional organisation to bring school nursing out of the cupboard and onto the community nursing agenda. What was identi-fied was a general lack of understanding among community nurse managers of the role of the school nurse (Bagnall, 1991). Orr (1991) emphasised the importance of developing standards for school nurses, and Bays (1991) discussed the importance of the effectiveness of programmes in enhancing the image of the school nurse. This raises the question of what would be useful outcome criteria. Two suggestions have been utilisation of the health services and student time lost from school (Jones and Clark, 1993).

Medicals or screening interviews

Until 1959, all children were required to have a medical inspection on entry to school. After that date, many health authorities offered a medical exami-nation to parents on a voluntary basis. Bolton (1994) described the replace-ment of the conventional school medical with a new system of screening school entrants by the school nurse in the Canterbury and Thanet health district. Not only was the system satisfactory to children and parents, but it also increased the school nurses' job satisfaction and was said to be more cost-effective. Houghton et al. (1992) proposed a similar system following a detailed study of 82 consecutive examinations performed by four school doctors on children aged over five. In Ealing, the health interview is the key part of the process of identifying children with health needs for medical examination and is conducted on all primary school entrants. The new programme not only releases school nurse time for developing health promo-tion activities within the core curriculum, but also acknowledges the impor-tant lead role of the school nurse within the school health service (Mattock, 1991). The objection to routine school medicals, including those for school leavers, generally concerns their cost-effectiveness in view of the small number of new problems that are detected (Roberts, 1993).

Current workload and training needs

Many authors have described the size of the case load. In Norwich, the case-load for individual nurses ranged from 400 to 1,500 pupils (Hawes, 1989). Adams (1992) reports on the workload of a particular school nurse in the school system in the USA who covers 2,500 pupils in one high school, one junior high school and three elementary schools.

Increasing activity has usually been accompanied by a large increase in the amount of clerical work, which is equally true when there is an increase in health education and health promotion (Nelson, 1989). Hunter (1991) studied the variety of tasks by using a diary of activities during a one-week period and concluded that routine tasks were getting in the way of others, such as health promotion, which might be more productive. This same point was made by Kobokovich and Bonovich (1992) in relation to adolescent pregnancy prevention activities.

Districts that have established strong school nursing programmes have usually developed a strong commitment to continuing education (Hawes, 1989). In a period of change and development within the NHS, continuing education is perhaps even more important (Collis, 1991). Some authors have stressed the importance of including the technical aspects of care in the continuing education programmes of school nurses. The need to maintain a high level of clinical expertise results from the increased presence of medically complex students in schools (Fegly et al., 1993; Felton and Parsons, 1993). Whatever the level of training or of commitment, it is difficult to see how nurses can adequately meet needs when they have case loads of the current size.

Expanding aspects of the current job

There is a widely held view that certain interventions are needed within schools. The first relates to the recognition of signs and symptoms, and includes drugs and alcohol, anorexia and child neglect or abuse. Another expanding area relates to the caring role, and covers the clinical needs of children with chronic illness, the immediate needs of those who are injured, including during school games and athletics, and also the care of pregnant teenagers. The role as screener or immuniser has seen several new angles. Another development is that of researcher/epidemiologist.

Recognition of signs

One of the problem areas for schools and for nurses is that of drugs and alcohol. There are problems of recognition of the signs and symptoms of substance use and a general lack of knowledge on how to manage overdose situations. One aid may be a nursing assessment tool that has been developed to identify students who may be using drugs or alcohol. It may identify students who need immediate medical care as well as those who are impaired by substance use but medically stable (Cromwell and LeMoine, 1992). Following a survey of cases referred from schools to a regional poisons centre, it appears that school nurses are not well prepared to recognise problems and are inadequately trained to deal with them (Perry et al., 1992).

Another problem area for early recognition is that of eating disorders. Anorexia nervosa is identified with increasing frequency among adolescents, and school nurses can play an important role in its primary, secondary and tertiary prevention. Connolly and Corbett (1990) propose a case management role for school nurses and consider that school nurses are uniquely placed to address these disorders. The school physician and the school nurse have special opportunities to detect situations of distress in children (Mantz, 1990). The importance of recognising neglect and intervening with these children's families is an essential element of the role of the school nurse. In a more recent study, school nurses were found to be extremely important in listening to young people's worries and concerns (Lightfoot and Bines, 2000).

The caring role

Given the increasing number of children with chronic disease who attend mainstream schools, it is inevitable that the school nurse will be increasingly involved in supporting their medical needs (Joachim, 1989; Repetto and Hoeman, 1991). Some of the conditions, for example asthma, are common. In an intervention study, Hill et al. (1991) set out to determine whether a programme based on existing school and community resources could reduce school absence and improve participation in games lessons and sport in children with unrecognised asthma. Teachers were given education on asthma by the school nurses.

Other conditions are rarely seen. Cooper (1989) gave an account of the key role of a school nurse for a child with a tracheotomy. One of the many issues that school nurses have to face is that of school-age pregnancy, which may involve providing antenatal support to young women at school (Chen et al., 1991).

Screening and immunisation

The literature on the role of school nurses in relation to immunisation will have to be rewritten following their involvement in the mass measles/rubella campaign in November 1994. Anecdotal evidence suggests that school nurses were central to the programme's overall success. Their role in

Canada's largest mass immunisation programme has been described by Bernatchez et al. (1993). In schools in North America, nurses play a pivotal role in the ascertainment of the appropriate immunisation status of school-children. One of the long-standing issues has been whether a doctor should or should not be present at the time the nurse gives the immunisation (Saffin, 1992).

On the screening side, there have been calls for the application of many different screening programmes, few of which have properly assessed their effectiveness. One proposal suggested the school nurse has a role in the detection of abnormal colour perception as well as in the education and counselling of affected students, their parents and their teachers (Evans, 1992).

Researcher and epidemiologist

Nurses are, in some cases, the developing focus for research into the health status and health problems of children. Several authors now see them as a key part of the research team. If school nurses become involved in systematic measurement, this raises the question of the reliability and validity of such measurements (Kelsall and Watson, 1990; Parker, 1992; Majrowski et al., 1994).

Health promotion opportunities

In this final section, consideration will be given to the school nurse's current role in health promotion and the constraints on and possibility of enlarging that role. There is an extensive opportunity to introduce health promotion as part of the curriculum. For school nurses to develop as the key figures in the school health service, they must broaden their role as health educators and health promoters (Johnson, 1991; DoH, 1992; Neylon, 1993; British Paediatric Association, 1995).

It has been widely recognised that teachers do not feel adequately prepared for sex education programmes. This issue was studied by Jackson (1989) in a study of all of the secondary schools and four special schools in Halton. Given teachers' general discomfiture, it is even more important that school nurses should be well trained in and comfortable with discussing sex education. An important issue is the age at which sex education should begin in schools. The prevailing view is that education about AIDS and HIV should start in primary school if positive attitudes and behaviour are to be effectively encouraged (Mole, 1991).

One aspect of health promotion is the provision of information. This applies to both the children themselves and to their parents. Patterson (1990) described how a request for health information from the mothers of young children led to a regular discussion group and a successful partnership between the school nurse and her health visitor colleagues.

In the climate of health service market orientation, purchasers were required to separate the specification of health promotion and health education from its delivery. The actual organisation of health promotion differs in different districts. In some it is an integral part of the district public health department, in others it is quasi independent, whereas in others it is a part of or an entirely separate legal entity. Examples include being part of a Trust or local authority.

Health educators have usually employed a combination of direct contact with individuals (children) and indirect contact through other health and educational professionals. In many districts, the absolute size of the health promotion and health education group is so small that it is difficult for them to function successfully even if they aspire only to an indirect role. For this role to be successful, health educators must develop a close working relationship with other health professionals. An obvious candidate is the school nurse. School nurses recognise that opportunity is not enough on its own but needs to be accompanied by well-developed programmes and policies. In many districts, the relationship between the health promotion specialist and the school nurse is close, contacts being frequent. In some, substantial time has been set aside for the development of the school nurse role. A World Health Organization study on health behaviour in schoolchildren described the pupils, the experience and the association with age, sex, geographical area and social class (Borup, 1998).

Health promotion constraints

Constraints remain much the same as before, depending to some extent on the imagination of the school nurse in accepting the challenge that others are grasping. The limitations rest largely on the climate of health service reforms, which have seen a substantial increase in the counting of activity and an increase in the political importance of acute hospital activity. The emphasis here is on waiting lists, hospital beds and day case surgery. Again, the school is relatively invisible, and the methods of counting the community nursing service in general and school nursing activities in particular is poorly developed.

When purchasers demand cost improvements in the budgets of community services, this may well mean a reduction in the number of school nurses. It requires a strong school nursing service to survive within a community Trust and a strong public health department at purchaser level to advocate its survival. In future, when GPs have an increasing say in how the health authority budget is to be spent, they are likely to be less sympathetic than those who currently take decisions about financial allocation.

Given the preference for the market testing of health and social services, as well as for the movement into the independent sector of some health and educational provision, school health services and school nursing services may be casualties in their current form. If the next decade is to see the survival of the school nursing service, it will be because of the recognition of its value by children and their parents (Lightfoot et al., 1998). Although their voices currently have only a minor influence on such policy decisions, it is not inconceivable that these voices will become louder.

If lessons from the USA teach us anything, it is that the school nursing service will disappear in many places, and re-creating it may not be easy. The challenge for school nurses is to grasp the many opportunities that exist. They must so enthuse about the school system, the children, the parents and the governors that those who take funding decisions will acknowledge the system's high profile and potential worth. The fact that the demonstration of effectiveness may be difficult in the short or medium term should not detract from the fact that there are many opportunities for instant feedback and visible success. Given the importance of their function, a key question is how to provide the most appropriate professional input (McDonald et al., 1997). The recent NHS consultation document on workforce planning is looking towards nurse professionals with a higher level of skills as well as general skills across a wider range of community nursing (Hargadon and Stainforth, 2000).

References

Adams, C.E. (1990) Perceptions of the comprehensive-based school nurse. *Health Visitor*, 63(3): 90–2.

Adams, C.E. (1991) An analysis of school nurse leadership styles. *Journal of School Nursing*, 7(2): 22–5.

Adams, C.E. (1992) Identification and recovery of co-dependent school nurses. *Journal of School Nursing*, 8(2): 14–15, 18–19.

Bagnall, P. (1989) School nursing: time to face the future. *Health Visitor*, 62(7): 224.

Bagnall, P. (1991) School nursing comes of age. *Health Visitor*, 64(5): 146–7.

Bagnall, P. and Dilloway, M. (1996a) *In a Different Light: School Nurses and their Role in Meeting the Needs of School Age Children*. London: DoH/Queen's Nursing Institute.

Bagnall, P. and Dilloway, M. (1996b) *In Search of a Blueprint: A Survey of School Health Services*. London: DoH/Queen's Nursing Institute.

Barnfather, J.S. (1991) Restructuring the role of the school nurse in health promotion. *Public Health Nurse*, 8(4): 234–8.

Bays, C.T. (1991) The school nurse: enhancing professional recognition. *Journal of School Nursing*, 7(3): 18–20, 22–4.

Bernatchez, M., Grakist, D., Lachance, M. et al. (1993) Operation Meningo: public health nurses' role in Canada's largest mass immunisation program. *Journal of School Health*, 63(10): 434–7.

Bolton, P. (1994) School entry screening by the school nurse. *Health Visitor*, 67(4): 135–6.

Borup, I.K. (1998) Pupils' experiences of the annual health dialogue with the school health nurse. *Scandinavian Journal of Caring Science*, **12**(3): 160–9.

British Paediatric Association (1995) *Health Needs of School Age Children*. London: BPA.

Brother, N. (1998) School nursing and student assistance: a natural partnership. *Journal of School Nursing*, **14**(1): 32–5.

Chen, S.P., Fitzgerald, M.C., DeStefano, L.M. and Chen, E.H. (1991) *Public Health Nurse*, **8**(4): 212–18.

Cohen, P. (1994) The role of the school nurse in providing sex education. *Nursing Times*, **90**(23): 36–8.

Collis, J. (1991) Education. What school nurses want. *Health Visitor*, **64**(5): 160–1.

Connolly, C. and Corbett, D.P. (1990) Eating disorders: a framework for school nursing initiatives. *Journal of School Health*, **60**(8): 401–5.

Cooper, H. (1989) Tracheostomy care in an educational setting. *Health Visitor*, **62**(Nov): 348–9.

Cromwell, P. and LeMoine, A. (1992) Identifying substance use: an assessment tool for the school nurse. *Journal of School Nursing*, **8**(3): 6–10, 12, 14–15.

DeBell, D. and Everett, G. (1997) *In a Class Apart: A Study of School Nursing*. Norwich: Research Centre, City College.

Department of Health (1992) *The Health of the Nation: A Strategy for Health in England*. London: HMSO.

Department of Health (1996) *Child Health in the Community: A Guide to Good Practice*. London: NHS Executive.

Department of Health (1997) *The New NHS: Modern, Dependable*. London: Stationery Office.

Department of Health (1998) *Saving Lives: Our Healthier Nation*. London: Stationery Office.

Doggett, M.A., Faulkner, A., Farrow, S. and Shelley, A. (1992) School nurses: constraints and opportunities for the future. *Journal of the Royal Society of Health*, **112**(2): 84–7.

Dolan, R., Corber, S. and Zacour, R. (1990) A survey of knowledge and attitudes with regard to AIDS among grade 7 and 8 students in Ottawa-Carleton. *Canadian Journal of Public Health*, **81**(2): 135–8.

Evans, A. (1992) Colour vision deficiency – what does it matter? *Journal of School Nursing*, **8**(4): 6–10.

Fegly, B.J., Wessel, G.L. and Diehl, B.C. (1993) Clinical continuing education for school nurses. *Journal of School Nursing*, **9**(3): 13–14, 16.

Felton, G.M. and Parsons, M.A. (1993) Improving school nursing practice in South Carolina through continuing education. *Journal of School Nursing*, **63**(5): 207–9.

Gaffrey, E.A. and Bergren, M.D. (1998) School health services and managed care: a unique partnership for child health. *Journal of School Health*, **14**(4): 14–20.

Greenhill, E.D. (1979) Perception of the school nurse's role. *Journal of School Health*, (Sep): 368–71.

Hacker, K. and Wessel, G.I. (1998) School-based health centres and school nurses: cementing the collaboration. *Journal of School Nursing*, **68**(10): 409–14.

Hansen, L. (1987) No longer the nit lady. *Nursing Times*, (3 Jun): 30–2.

Hargadon, J. and Stainforth, M. (2000) *A Health Service of All the Talents: Developing the NHS Workforce*. Consultation document on the review of workforce planning. Department of Health 1P.25K.APRIL 2000. (CWP) 21325. London: DoH.

Harrison, A. and Gretton, J. (1986) School health: the invisible service. In *Health Care UK, An Economic, Social and Policy Audit.* Hermitage: Policy Journals: 25–32.

Hawes, M. (1989) School nursing in Norwich Health Authority. *Health Visitor,* 62(11): 351–2.

Health Visitors Association (1988) *Meeting Schoolchilden's Health Needs.* London: HVA.

Health Visitors Association (1996) *School Nursing: Here Today for Tomorrow.* London: HVA.

Hill, R., Williams, J., Britton, J. and Tattersfield, A. (1991) Can morbidity associated with untreated asthma in primary school children be reduced?: a controlled intervention study. *British Medical Journal,* 303(6811): 1169–74.

Houghton, A., Ean, S., Archibal, G., Bradley, O. and Azam, N. (1992) Selective medical examination at school entry: should we do it, and if so how? *Journal of Public Health Medicine,* 14(2): 111–16.

Hunter, A. (1991) A week in the life of Alice Hunter. *Health Visitor,* 664(5): 162–3.

Igoe, J.B. (1994) School nursing. *Nursing Clinics of North America,* 29(3): 443–58.

Jackson, C. (1991) Turning back the clock. *Health Visitor,* 64(5): 148–9.

Jackson, C. (1992) Swings and roundabouts. *Health Visitor,* 65(11): 392–3.

Jackson, D. (1989) Sex education in Halton secondary schools. *Health Visitor,* 62: 219–21.

Joachim, G. (1989) The school nurse as case manager for chronically ill children. *Journal of School Health,* 59(9): 406–7.

Johnson, J. (1991) Classroom health promotion. *Health Visitor,* 64(5): 152–3.

Jones, M.E. and Clark, D. (1993) What school nurses really do – a study of school nurse utilisation. *Journal of School Nursing,* 9(2): 10–17.

Juhn, G., Tang, J., Piessens, P. et al. (1999) Community learning: the reach of the health nursing program–middle school collaboration. *Journal of Nursing Education,* 38(5): 215–21.

Kelsall, J.E. and Watson, A.R. (1990) Should school nurses measure blood pressure. *Public Health,* 104(3): 191–4.

Klahn, L.K., Hays, B.J. and Iverson, C.J. (1998) The school health intensity scale: establishing reliability for practice. *Journal of School Nursing,* 14(4): 23–8.

Kobokovich, L.J. and Bonovich, L.K. (1992) Adolescent pregnancy prevention strategies used by school nurses. *Journal of School Health,* 62(1): 11–14.

Lightfoot, J. and Bines W. (2000) Working to keep school children healthy: the complementary roles of school staff and school nurses. *Journal of Public Health Medicine,* 22(1): 74–80.

Lightfoot, J., Wright, S. and Sloper, P. (1998) *Service Support for Children with Chronic Illness or Physical Disability Attending Mainstream Schools.* York: Social Policy Research Unit, University of York.

Lochhead, E. (1994) Introducing nursery nurses to the school health team. *Health Visitor,* 67(4): 133–4.

McDonald, A.L., Langford, I.H. and Boldero, N. (1997) The future of community nursing in the United Kingdom: district nursing, health visiting and school nursing. *Journal of Advanced Nursing,* 26(2): 257–65.

Majrowski, W.H., Hearn, S., Rohan, C. et al. (1994) Comparison of school nurse and auxologist height velocity measurements in school children with short stature. *Child Care Health Development,* 20(3): 179–83.

Mantz, J. (1990) The school physician and the abused child. *Annals of Pediatrics (Paris),* 37(2): 123–6.

Mattock, C. (1991) Health interviews. Stepping off the medical treadmill. *Health Visitor*, **64**(5): 154–6.

Mole, S. (1991) AIDS education in schools. *Health Visitor*, **64**(7): 221–2.

National Association of State School Nurse Consultants (1993) A position statement of the National Association of State School Nurse Consultants. Medicaid reimbursement for school nursing services, August. *Journal of School Nursing*, **9**(3): 37–9.

Nelson, M. (1989) The changing role of the school nurse within Worcester and District Health Authority. *Health Visitor*, **62**: 349–50.

Neylon, J. (1993) School nursing: health promotion for school children. *Nursing Standard*, 7(30): 37–40.

Orr, J. (1991) Valuing school nurses. *Health Visitor*, **64**(5): 147.

Parker, S.H. (1992) The school nurse's role: early detection of growth disorders. *Journal of School Nursing*, **8**(3): 30–2, 34, 36–8.

Parsons, M.A. and Felton, G.M. (1992) Role performance and job satisfaction of school nurses. *Western Journal of Nursing Research*, **14**(4): 498–511.

Patterson, A. (1990) A school nurse and health visitor working together as health educators. *Health Visitor*, **63**(11): 391.

Perry, P.A., Dean, B.S. and Krenzelok, E.P. (1992) A regional poison centre's experience with poisoning exposures occurring in schools. *Veterinary and Human Toxicology*, **34**(2): 148–51.

Primary Health Care Group (1988) *Changing School Health Service*. London: King's Fund Centre for Health Services Development.

Repetto, M.A. and Hoeman, S.P. (1991) A legislative perspective on the school nurse and education for children with disabilities in New Jersey. *Journal of School Nursing*, **61**(9): 388–91.

Roberts, P.J. (1993) The school leaver medical: and evaluation. *Public Health*, **107**(2): 113–16.

Saffin, K. (1992) School nurses immunising without a doctor present. *Health Visitor*, **65**(11): 394–6.

Staunton, P. (1983) Images of the primary school nurse. *Nursing Times*, (31 Aug): 49–52.

Thompson, J. (1989) School health services in the United States: a view from the United Kingdom. *Journal of School Health*, **59**(6): 243–5.

Thurber, F., Berry, B. and Cameron, M.E. (1991) The role of school nursing in the United States. *Journal of Pediatric Health Care*, **5**(3): 135–40.

Thyer, S. (1996) The 'health promoting schools" strategy: implications for nursing and allied health professionals. *Collegian* (Journal of the Royal College of Nursing, Australia), **3**(2): 13–23.

Turner, T. (1994) A message for Mrs Bottomley. *Health Visitor*, **67**(4): 121–2.

While, A.E. and Barriball, K.L. (1993) School nursing: history, present practice and possibilities reviewed. *Journal of Advanced Nursing*, **18**(8): 1202–11.

Yates, S.R. (1992) The school nurse's role: early intervention with preschool children. *Journal of School Nursing*, **8**(4): 30–6.

CHAPTER 14

Health-promoting Universities: An Overview

MARK DOORIS AND JANE THOMPSON

During the past decade, an increasing number of universities have taken an interest in developing a range of health promotion activities focused on students and staff. A smaller number have drawn on the settings-based approach to develop more strategic and comprehensive, whole-organisation health-promoting initiatives for universities and colleges. This chapter offers an overview of the settings-based approach to health promotion, considers the characteristics that make university and college settings distinctive, provides a case study of the Health-promoting University (HPU) initiative at Central Lancashire and discusses key issues facing professionals involved in developing and implementing health-promoting university and college initiatives.

The settings-based approach to health promotion

The concept of health-promoting universities has emerged as part of what has become known as settings-based health promotion. Health promotion has focused on settings for many years, most commonly in terms of carrying out health promotion, or more often health education, *within* particular settings. The concept of a settings-based approach has, however, developed more recently. It is widely accepted that its roots lie within the new public health movement (WHO, 1998a), more specifically within the World Health Organization (WHO) Health for All strategy (WHO, 1980, 1985, 1998b) and the Ottawa Charter for Health Promotion (WHO, 1986). The latter drew upon both Health for All and the work of theorists concerned with the creation of positive health, what Antonovsky (1987, 1996) has called salutogenic research, representing a critical point in the emergence of the settings-based approach. Reflecting a growing consensus that health is a socio-ecological product that can be developed most effectively and efficiently by investing *outside* the healthcare sector, the Ottawa Charter stated that:

> Health is created and lived by people within the settings of their everyday life; where they learn, work, play and love. Health is created by caring for oneself and others, by being able to take decisions and have control over one's life circum-

stances, and by ensuring that the society one lives in creates conditions that allow the attainment of health by all its members. (WHO, 1986: iii–v)

The Ottawa Charter served as a catalyst to shift health promotion away from problems characterised by particular behaviours or specific at-risk groups, towards environments and settings. It adopted a fivefold focus on healthy public policy, the creation of environments supportive to health, strengthening community action, developing personal skills and reorienting health services. This holistic environmental focus was strengthened by the subsequent publication of a number of documents from the WHO (1990, 1991, 1992, 1994a, 1994b), being further reinforced by the 1992 United Nations Earth Summit as well as the resulting Rio Declaration (United Nations, 1992) and Agenda 21 (United Nations, 1993), which highlighted the growing convergence of sustainable development and health agenda.

The first and best-known example of settings-based health promotion is the Healthy Cities strategy, which started as a small WHO project in 1986 and rapidly grew to become a major global movement (Tsouros, 1991). The late 1980s and early 1990s saw parallel initiatives take root in a number of smaller settings such as schools (Rasmussen and Rivett, 2000) and hospitals (Tsouros, 1993), as well as, within the UK, the endorsement of the settings-based approach through government policy (DoH, 1992, 1999).

As Dooris et al. (1998) have argued, it is possible to draw upon and synthesise ideas from a number of theorists and practitioners (Baric, 1993, 1994; Grossman and Scala, 1993; Dowding, 1995; Harrison, 1995; Kickbusch, 1995; White and Bhopal, 1995; Dooris, 1998) to outline the key characteristics of the settings-based approach to health promotion: First, the following underpinning principles and perspectives can be identified, drawn largely from Health for All, the Ottawa Charter and Agenda 21:

- a holistic, socio-ecological model of health;
- consensus and mediation;
- equity and social justice;
- advocacy;
- sustainability;
- settings as part of an interdependent ecosystem;
- participation;
- a focus on the setting as a social system;
- enablement and empowerment;
- a focus on populations, policy and environments;
- cooperation;
- a commitment to sustainable integrative actions.

Second, the settings-based approach is characterised by the use of particular processes and techniques, drawn from management, organisation and systems theory. Through organisational development, it is possible to identify why and how a healthy organisation can perform better and how a commitment to and an investment in health can be embedded within the structures, mechanisms, culture and routine life of the institution. In turn, organisational development can be most effectively instituted through the use of project management, concerned with the processes of change management, policy development, knowledge and skills development, and quality, audit and evaluation.

Third, Baric (1994) has argued that the settings-based approach is characterised by three key elements:

1. creating a healthy working and living environment, for example through ensuring supportive management styles, employment practices and social and recreational opportunities;

2. integrating health promotion into the daily activities of the setting, for example through focusing on its routine life and considering how organisational development techniques can embed health within this;

3. reaching out into the wider community, for example through building partnerships and alliances, providing resources, considering the impact of the settings-based approach on the local, national and global communities, purchasing, financial management and other practices, practising advocacy and mediation roles, and so on.

Applying the settings-based approach within higher education

Universities have not been mentioned specifically in government health policy, but there is growing interest in exploring the application of the settings-based approach within this sector. This is fuelled by both interest within health promotion and public health, and an increased focus within education, on quality and excellence. Universities have a number of functions common to any large organisation, but they also have roles that create distinctive characteristics and cultures. These include:

- a focus on education, training and research;
- a role in developing as centres of creativity and innovation, combining, managing and applying ideas and processes within and between disciplines;
- providing a setting in which students of all ages can develop intellectually and personally, often by experimenting and by exploring what sort of person they hope to become;
- acting as a resource for communities and agencies, locally, nationally or globally;
- succeeding as a financial enterprise (Abercrombie, 1998).

Most of these roles create opportunities for developing health as a value and a practical resource. One of the most valuable roles for a health-promoting university or college is perhaps to become an advocate for developing healthy public policy at both local and national level. There are, however, also challenges, shaped largely by national policy and trends.

A series of funding cuts combined with a strategy to increase student numbers, particularly of part-time and non-traditional students, have left staff with an increased and changing workload. There is a pressure on staff to obtain higher degrees and to be actively involved in research and publishing, very often securing the funding for this, but with little or no extra time made available. The effect is that many staff are working longer hours and reporting an increased level of stress and reduced job satisfaction (Association of University Teachers, 1994).

Students, too, are under greater pressure to combine study with paid employment, to be actively seeking a future career in a changing and volatile job market and to negotiate their way through a college or university system in which libraries, other resources and staff provision may all be underfunded (Abercrombie, 1998).

Overall, however, there is a significant potential for universities, out of all settings, to develop and demonstrate the core values that are intrinsic to a health-promoting organisation, namely democracy, empowerment, autonomy and community participation (Simnett, 1995).

A case study: University of Central Lancashire

In 1995, the University of Central Lancashire became one of the first universities in Europe to establish an HPU initiative. The roots of the initiative can be traced back to 1992, when the university was instrumental in Preston being selected as the English pilot within the WHO European Health-promoting Hospital project. An international seminar on the settings-based approach to health promotion, subsequently organised by the university in collaboration with the WHO and the North West Regional Health Authority, led to a growing interest in applying the approach within the institution itself. This interest was nurtured by the progressive Department of Health Studies within a broad-based Faculty of Health, resulting in two years' faculty research monies being allocated to fund a full-time post comprising a half-time Lecturer in Health Studies and a half-time HPU Coordinator.

The first task was to develop a conceptual framework that would enable the settings-based approach to be applied within the university. This required both a review of the literature referred to above and extensive networking with key departments, services and external bodies to gain a clear understanding of what was in place, what gaps there were and what characterised the organisational context, as well as to build support among stakeholders. Guided by the principles, perspectives, processes and elements characterising the settings-based approach outlined above, it was agreed that the overarching aims of the HPU initiative should be:

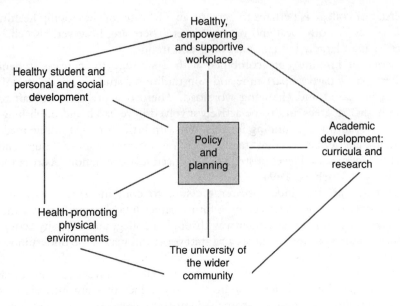

Figure 14.1   Agenda for action

- to integrate, within the university's culture, processes and structures, a commitment to health and to developing its health-promoting potential;
- to promote the health and well-being of staff, students and the wider community.

Within these overall aims, six objectives were set, forming a broad agenda for action (Figure 14.1):

- to integrate a commitment to and vision of health within the university's plans and policies;
- to support the healthy personal and social development of students;
- to develop the university as a supportive, empowering and healthy workplace;
- to create health-promoting and sustainable physical environments;
- to increase understanding, knowledge and the commitment to multidisciplinary health promotion across all university faculties and departments;
- to support the promotion of sustainable health in the wider community.

The term 'sustainable health' was chosen to emphasise two facets of effective health promotion: first, a recognition that health is dependent upon environmentally and socially sustainable human development, as articulated within Agenda 21 (United Nations, 1993); and second, a concern to ensure that health promotion interventions are themselves durable and sustainable in the way in which they are set up and implemented.

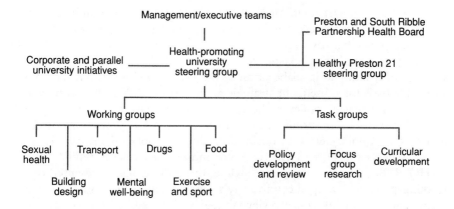

Figure 14.2 Organisational structure

Having agreed a conceptual framework and gained basic support for the initiative, the next task was to establish an appropriate organisational structure able to oversee the initiative's implementation. A senior-level steering group was set up that could establish working groups and short-term sub-groups as necessary, with clear reporting and accountability routes and links to parallel internal and external committees and partnerships (Figure 14.2).

The working groups were set up over a period of time in response to identified need, interest and motivation, harnessing and focusing enthusiasm and available resources, and utilising real-life entry points within the constraints of the existing organisational culture. The first four priority focus areas – sexual health, building design, transport and mental well-being – were not only important in their own right, but also served to reflect and articulate the HPU's breadth of vision. Subsequent areas prioritised have included drugs, food, and exercise and sport.

Drawing on the WHO's experience in developing its Healthy Cities Project, the work of the steering group and the working groups has sought to build managerial commitment and widespread ownership, as well as to combine the coordination of high-visibility activities for health with innovative action and long-term organisational development and institutional change (Tsouros, 1991; Tsouros et al., 1998). An overview of some of the work carried out in pursuit of the six overlapping objectives identified in the agenda for action, serves to illustrate this approach and highlight some key achievements.

The policy process

Integrating a commitment to and a vision of health within the routine policy-making and planning cycles of the university is central to the initiative. The adoption by the university in March 1997 of a corporate policy on health was seen as a natural first step, building as it did upon the university's strongly developed policy framework.

The articulation of a holistic approach, in relation to both its under-standing of health and its elaboration of the HPU's objectives, has served as a valuable basis for subsequent strategic action via the dual routes of moving from a health-specific policy to healthy policies in general, and developing focused guidance on specific health issues. The former, whereby health becomes a central criterion in decision making and policy development as a whole, reflects the Ottawa Charter's commitment to healthy public policy (WHO, 1986). Positive steps here include the HPU being represented on a working party reviewing the university's mission statement, and the agree-ment that subsequent policy review should seek to embed the concept of sustainable health within the university's overall planning and policy frame-work. Ways of increasing participation and transparency in decision-making processes are also to be considered.

One area in which specific guidelines have been formulated and adopted is that of drugs. These were prioritised because of a concern about the lack of clear guidance on how to respond to drug-related incidents. Following consultative training, guidelines were developed by a multi-agency task group, taking account of and balancing the full range of legal, welfare, educational, health and safety, and professional conduct/customer care responsibilities.

Student development

This leads onto the second priority area, concerned with supporting the healthy personal and social development of students, in ways that reflect the HPU's concern with enabling students to explore and develop an under-standing of themselves as whole people and to empower them to develop their full potential. Such an approach requires a substantial investment in supportive structures, systems and processes, as well as a willingness to innovate.

Through working in active cooperation with student services, the students' union and the student accommodation services to promote well-being, the HPU has tried to build upon the university's existing commitment to such investment in relation to general service provision and specific topics such as sexual health. One example of innovation is Touch, a multi-disciplinary and multi-agency peer education and outreach project focusing on sexual health promotion and safer drug use within the setting of Feel, one of the UK's top student club nights. The project has achieved high visibility and sustainability, and is characterised by the use of indigenous volunteering, harm-reduction approaches and value-free information. Following its successful establishment and consolidation, the feasibility of developing an academic module in health-focused peer education is being explored.

Supportive, empowering and healthy workplace

Third, there is a commitment to developing the university as a supportive, empowering and healthy workplace. In the same way that support systems are crucial to sustaining student well-being, supportive staffing procedures and services are a cornerstone upon which the HPU has sought to build a further commitment to a healthy and empowering workplace. One of the key planks of this work has been the gradual bringing together of different services to focus on workplace health, particularly mental well-being. This has resulted in a growing synergy between personnel services, health and safety and the HPU initiative as a whole. This synergy was most recently characterised by management-level discussions on the development of a policy statement and an organisational action plan on stress and mental well-being, which, it is anticipated, will recognise and address the interface between staff and student health.

A specific project carried out in 1999 was the production of men's and women's health handbooks aimed at enabling both individual self-skilling and self-help, as well as at empowering staff and students to work for and advocate organisational change. The decision to produce common handbooks was taken in recognition of the demographic overlaps between, and the value of challenging existing stereotypes of, students and staff. The two handbooks were researched and written by journalism graduates who had represented the students' union on the HPU Steering Group. This decision reflected the HPU ethos of encouraging personal development and empowerment, the process being overseen by an experienced health promotion journalist and an inter-departmental and multi-agency advisory group. The two booklets list common health issues, give general information and practical tips, and include phone numbers and Web site addresses.

Supportive and health-promoting physical environments

There is a recognition that the quality of the physical environment affects the health and well-being of people, and a consequent commitment to create environments that are sustainable and supportive to health. In support of the HPU, a virtual working group, led by the department of property services, has explored ways in which new-build and refurbishment schemes can integrate a range of green and health-enhancing features. Furthermore, there has been a strong commitment to developing a green, visually attractive and safe campus. All of these features contribute to promoting and sustaining holistic health.

A further working group has focused on transport, encouraging and enabling the use of alternatives to the car and working with other agencies to develop a draft green transport plan. There is still a long way to go, and the process has not been without its obstacles, but at least the issues are on the agenda and some progress has been made.

Academic development

Finally, there is a commitment to increasing the understanding of, and competencies in, health through academic development, embedding health within the curriculum. A task group has met to explore possible ways forward, highlighting the importance of a number of specific areas. Collaboration with a key skills project has enabled the exploration of the role of the educational process in enabling the development of key transferable skills and competencies for life. These skills empower students to take increased control over their health and equip them to achieve their full potential in and outside work as individuals, citizens and members of communities.

The potential both for an awareness and understanding of health and competencies, and for health promotion to be integrated into and across a diversity of disciplines and professional training, has been explored in small-scale ways. This has contributed to awareness raising within the university, as, for example, with photography students producing installations for World AIDS Day, and potentially strengthening students' commitment to health in their future lives.

Health of the wider community

There is a concern to promote health within the wider community, which has been developed in two main ways; through working in partnership with other agencies and through providing resources for people living in Preston and the region. Formal partnership working, such as the Healthy Preston 21 initiative, has ensured that health issues are viewed within a broad context and resources and energy are effectively harnessed and channelled. Informal partnerships, such as the World AIDS Day Angel Quilts project, brought together many people from the local community who had never previously ventured into the university, to work alongside staff, students and local health workers.

With regard to serving as a local resource, the university, through its well-developed access routes, has long viewed itself as an educational resource for the community. Beyond this, it also offers many of its recreational and cultural facilities to the wider community, examples being students' union and arts centre events, as well as the new outdoor sports arena, opened in April 2000. All of these commitments, although they cannot strictly speaking be labelled 'health', make an important contribution to well-being.

Professional perspectives: key issues involved in developing and implementing health-promoting university and college initiatives

The overview above highlights a range of achievements and points to the potential value of applying settings-based health promotion within universities.

An evaluation of the first phase of the Central Lancashire initiative (Dooris, 1998) indicated success in achieving the short-term objectives. There was a growing recognition of the HPU's potential to increase the well-being of staff, students and the wider community, as well as, more broadly, to add value to the university in terms of overall distinctiveness, performance and productivity.

There were, however, challenges, and it is useful to highlight some key issues that can face the professionals involved in establishing and developing initiatives:

- *Organisational base.* A key issue is where to locate a project. Different universities have chosen different bases, and there is no one right answer. An academic department may, for example, offer the advantage of enabling curricular links and adding legitimacy to the project, while student services or human resources/occupational health may help to mainstream the project but may also create a perception that the only focus is on either students or staff.

- *Implementing 'holistic health'.* It is apparent from the above summary that even though the perspective adopted was holistic, it proved necessary to break health down into a number of easily digestible parts, such as staff health, student health and curriculum, or sexual health, mental well-being and transport. The experience of Central Lancashire is that it is possible, over time, to develop an understanding of the ecological nature of health and forge links between working groups.

- *Project-ism.* For the first few years of Central Lancashire's initiative, people viewed it as a discrete project, interesting, even important, but definitely someone else's (the coordinator's) responsibility. A challenge to any new initiative is to move from being seen as a separate project to being understood as a mainstream initiative involving a wide range of services and faculties as responsible actors.

- *Perspectives.* As in any setting, those professionals coordinating an initiative in a university or college will confront different perspectives on health promotion – not least the view that it should be about only individual responsibility and self-help. The settings-based approach, rooted as it is in the understanding that health can only be meaningfully promoted if individual and community action is underpinned and supported by organisational development and change, requires that such perspectives be challenged. Advocating that health promotion should focus on such areas as management style, communication systems, decision-making procedures, workload, level of pay, student finance and job security is, however, likely to be uncomfortable. Mediation for health might be required, using language that taps into current concerns, be they student recruitment and retention, staff performance or legislature regarding stress.

- *Power relations.* Related to this is the challenge of combining a commitment to a top-down and bottom-up action, both being an essential part of a balanced and effective approach. It is important to build senior management commitment and to develop broad-based ownership by staff, students and the wider community, and combining these elements can be extremely challenging.

To conclude, universities occupy a unique position in seeking to practise and promote holistic health: they have not only the capacity to make changes to their institutional practice, but also a unique responsibility and potential to educate and influence the next generation of decision makers and managers. The Health-promoting University and College model provides an invaluable framework for promoting health and well-being in an integrated and far-reaching way that takes account of the relationships between environments and behaviours, as well as between staff, students and the wider community.

The WHO is committed to developing work in this field, its Healthy Cities Phase III Strategic Plan (WHO, 1998c) including, as a strategic priority, highlighting initiatives to promote health in the specific setting of cities, including the development of HPU projects.

The future establishment of a European initiative promises to be an exciting development and one that offers the opportunity for future cooperation and shared learning at both national and international level.

References

Abercrombie, N. (1998) Universities and health in the twenty-first century. In Tsouros, A., Dowding, G., Thompson, J. and Dooris, M. (eds) *Health Promoting Universities: Concept, Experience and Framework for Action.* Copenhagen: WHO.

Antonovsky, A. (1987) *Unraveling the Mystery of Health.* San Francisco: Jossey-Bass.

Antonovsky, A. (1996) The salutogenic model as a theory to guide health promotion. *Health Promotion International,* 11(1): 11–18.

Association of University Teachers (1994) *Long Hours, Little Thanks – a Survey of the Use of Time by Full-time Academic and Related Staff in the Traditional UK Universities.* London: AUT.

Baric, L. (1993) The settings approach – implications for policy and strategy. *Journal of the Institute of Health Education,* 31(1): 17–24.

Baric, L. (1994) *Health Promotion and Health Education in Practice: Module 2 – the Organisational Model.* Altrincham: Barns.

Department of Health (1992) *The Health of the Nation: A Strategy for Health in England.* London: HMSO.

Department of Health (1999) *Saving Lives: Our Healthier Nation.* London: Stationery Office.

Dooris, M. (1998) *Working for Sustainable Health: University of Central Lancashire Health Promoting University Phase I Progress and Evaluation Report.* Preston: University of Central Lancashire.

Dooris, M., Dowding, G., Thompson, J. and Wynne, C. (1998) The settings-based approach to health promotion. In Tsouros, A., Dowding, G., Thompson, J. and Dooris, M. (eds) *Health Promoting Universities: Concept, Experience and Framework for Action*. Copenhagen: WHO.

Dowding, G. (1995) *Health Promoting University Project: First Annual Report*. Lancaster: Morecambe Bay Health Promotion.

Grossman, R. and Scala, K. (1993) *Health Promotion and Organisational Development: Developing Settings for Health*. Copenhagen: WHO.

Harrison, D. (1995) Health Promoting Hospitals in Europe. In Riley, C., Warner, M., Semple Piggott, C. and Pullen, A. (eds) *Releasing Resources to Achieve Health Gain*. London: Routledge.

Kickbusch, I. (1995) An overview to the settings-based approach to health promotion. In Theaker, T. and Thompson, J. (eds) *The Settings-based Approach to Health Promotion: Conference Report*. Welwyn Garden City: Hertfordshire Health Promotion.

Rasmussen, V.B. and Rivett, D. (2000) The European network of health promoting schools – an alliance of health, education and democracy. *Health Education*, **100**(2): 61–7.

Simnett, I. (1995) *Managing Health Promotion: Developing Healthy Organisations and Communities*. London: John Wiley & Sons.

Tsouros, A. (ed.) (1991) *World Health Organization Healthy Cities Project: A Project Becomes a Movement. Review of Progress 1987–1990*. Copenhagen/Milan: FADL Publishers/SOGESS.

Tsouros, A. (1993) Health promoting hospitals: European perspectives. In Health Education Authority (ed.) *Health Promoting Hospitals: Principles and Practice*. London: HEA.

Tsouros, A., Dowding, G., Thompson, J. and Dooris, M. (eds) (1998) *Health Promoting Universities: Concept, Experience and Framework for Action*. Copenhagen: WHO.

United Nations (1992) *Rio Declaration on Environment and Development*. New York: UN.

United Nations (1993) *Earth Summit – Agenda 21*. New York: UN Department of Public Information.

White, M. and Bhopal, R. (1995) Health policy development in a medical school. *HFANews* (Faculty of Public Health Medicine of the Royal Colleges of Physicians), **31**: 6–9.

World Health Organization (1980) *European Regional Strategy for Health for All*. Copenhagen: WHO.

World Health Organization (1985) *Targets for Health for All*. Copenhagen: WHO.

World Health Organization (1986) Ottawa Charter for Health Promotion. *Health Promotion International*, **1**(4): iii–v.

World Health Organization (1990) *Environment and Health. The European Charter and Commentary*. Copenhagen: WHO.

World Health Organization (1991) *Sundsvall Statement on Supportive Environments for Health*. Geneva: WHO.

World Health Organization (1992) *Our Planet, Our Health: Report of the WHO Commission on Health and Environment*. Geneva: WHO.

World Health Organization (1994a) *Environmental Health Action Plan for Europe*. Copenhagen: WHO.

World Health Organization (1994b) *Declaration on Action for Environment and Health in Europe*. Copenhagen: WHO.

World Health Organization (1997) *Jakarta Declaration on Health Promotion into the 21st Century*. Copenhagen: WHO.

World Health Organization (1998a) *Health Promotion Glossary*. Geneva: WHO.

World Health Organization (1998b) *Health 21 – the Health for All Policy for the WHO European Region: 21 Targets for the 21st Century*. Copenhagen: WHO.

World Health Organization (1998c) *Strategic Plan: Urban Health/Healthy Cities Programme (1998–2002): Phase III of the WHO Healthy Cities Project*. Geneva: WHO.

CHAPTER 15

Health Promotion in Youth Work Settings

SUE ROBERTSON

Recent government initiatives, particularly the concentration on social exclusion, have put young people at the forefront of government policy in many different areas and impacted on the work of the youth service. A new government initiative, *Connexions* (DfEE, 2000a) proposes giving every young person the best start in life via various initiatives, including employing student mentors in schools and creating a new profession of personal advisers. The Policy Action Team (1999) report on young people, *Young People 2000*, proposes the creation of a youth unit to coordinate policy at both national and local level. Both *Young People 2000* and *Connexions* highlight the need for young people to be involved in policy development and in-service delivery, and for different agencies to work together. *Connexions*, for example, will be run by a partnership in each area.

Young (1999) depicts the youth service as one undergoing change while enjoying influence, its methods of informal education and its ability to contact and work alongside young people being commended. Youth workers are being included in partnership initiatives such as Youth Offending Teams, New Deal for Communities, Education Action Zones, Health Action Zones (Policy Action Team, 1999). *Saving Lives: Our Healthier Nation* (DoH, 1999) sets out targets for the reduction in the number of deaths from heart disease, accidents, mental health and cancer. *Tackling Drugs to Build a Better Britain* (Cabinet Office, 1998) and the Social Exclusion Unit teenage pregnancy report highlight the issues faced by many young people today. In all these areas, the health education of young people is vital, the youth service being involved in many different types of initiative throughout the country (see, for example, Harker et al., 1999). In reaching adolescents, youth workers generally recommend a holistic approach to health education that helps young people to make decisions and choices (Young, 1999), an approach described by Heaven (1996) as a biopsychosocial model.

With these new ways of working, it is, however, important that the youth service retains its unique professional role, based on a voluntary relationship with young people and grounded in generic work. The key purpose of youth work is to work with young people to facilitate their personal, social and educational development, enabling them to gain a voice, influence and place in society in a period of transition from dependence to independence (National Youth Agency, 2000). Youth work is largely engaged in the informal education of young people, with individuals and/or with groups, particularly but not exclusively with teenagers between the ages of 13 and 19. This stage in a young person's development is a time of critical transition from adolescence to adulthood, when young people are perhaps more urgently in need of knowledge and information about matters that affect their mental, emotional and physical health. As such, it is a primary period for health education.

Youth work takes place in a variety of settings. These include local authority youth clubs and centres, detached work projects, girls groups, sports clubs and youth advice and information centres, as well as voluntary organisation groups such as the Scouts, Guides, Woodcraft Folk, youth theatres, church youth groups and many other single-focus activity groups. These places offer young people an environment where they can feel safe and operate on their own terms with adults they know and trust. Youth workers, therefore, come from a range of backgrounds; some are full-time paid professionals with a recognised national qualification, whereas others may work one night a week as a paid locally qualified worker or give their time voluntarily.

Of enormous significance is the fact that young people participate in youth service activities voluntarily, choosing to attend rather than being compelled to do so, as they must school and formal education activities. Issues of equality of opportunity are also very important in youth work, many projects engaging with single-gender, gay and lesbian, disabled or ethnic groups, helping them to explore their identity. An important aim for youth workers is the empowerment of young people. They are encouraged to take control of their own youth project and to attempt to influence those with power around them. Many projects demonstrate the ability of young people to do this, as a recent conference organised and run by young people for youth workers and policy makers demonstrated (UK Youth, 2000).

The combination of factors outlined above makes youth work unique in educational terms. Young people take centre stage, engaging in chosen activities in their own free time, where they can feel safe with their peers and trusted adults, without external pressure. These informal settings offer a tremendous opportunity for health promotion, even regarding such basic matters as what to sell in the coffee bar, which posters to have on the walls, which information leaflets to provide and what conversations to have. The main tool of youth workers is conversation and the ability to lead it into important areas so that young people are able to identify and work on their own needs (Jeffs and Smith, 1996; Young, 1999). These may include health needs, which young people may choose to explore using activities and games, for example, or be helped to move on to more ambitious projects such as those described later in this chapter. Used well and sensitively, youth work presents an opportunity for health education work with young people that is often impossible to re-create in a more formal setting.

Accessing and involving young people

The potential of the youth service in promoting health with young people has generally been underutilised, much health-focused youth work going unaided and unrecognised. The National Youth Agency has called on the new Health Development Agency to acknowledge the contribution that youth work makes by evaluating the health gain to young people through such work (Beebee, 2000a).

A government survey by the Office of Population Censuses and Surveys (OPCS) included questions on young people's involvement with the youth service. Out of a total of 3,700 young people contacted in late 1993 and early 1994, this survey showed that 20 per cent of young people aged between 13 and 19 were participating in youth service activities (Department for Education, 1995). Extrapolated onto a national scale, this implies something in the order of 840,000 young people, not including the millions of under-11s involved in the junior wings of uniformed organisations or youth clubs. The researchers claimed the figures suggested that the youth service reached 63 per cent of young people at some time during their teenage years. Today, this would be a target population of approximately 2.7 million. The research also found that, of those aged between 11 and 25 who used the service, the majority used it extensively, some 1.13 million at least once each week.

The youth service has demonstrated, therefore, the voluntary engagement of a considerable number of young people at a period in their lives generally regarded in health terms as being important because lifestyle habits and behaviour are being established. Because of this, it should not be overlooked when health promotion initiatives are being formulated and healthy alliances promoted.

Interagency work

Some regional and district health authorities have recognised the potential impact that progressive and innovative youth projects can make and have provided funding (Bloxham, 1998). Bloxham's research examined interagency collaboration in the field of young people's sexual health. The findings indicate that, although youth and community workers had a distinctive role to play, this often went unrecognised by schools, health services and other agencies. Bloxham also suggests that youth service involvement may encourage other agencies to adopt a more empowering and inclusive response. The examples below show what can be accomplished in this way.

The Health Line Project was initiated to introduce health education into the youth service curriculum, by establishing a partnership between Liverpool Health Authority and Merseyside Youth Association, to deliver directly through youth clubs and to train youth workers to deliver their own programmes. It aims to raise young people's awareness of health issues, provides advice, helps people to access local health services and supports peer education programmes (Warnock, 1999). The Den in Duffryn Health Promotion Drop-In Centre in Newport, Wales is a drop-in health promotion and resource centre targeting young people and their parents (New Opportunities Fund, 1999). The centre opened in April 1996, funded by Gwent health authority and staffed by community and youth workers. The project contracts in health and other workers for services such as a young people's clinic, careers advice and a baby clinic. It also offers activities such as photography and is striving to be user led.

These projects offer practical examples of provision that has been shown to work, as well as of dynamic partnerships between health professionals and the youth service. Another example is based at Paignton Community College in Devon, where a youth worker coordinates a multi-disciplinary team funded by the health authority, including general practitioners (GPs), nurses and health visitors, to run a project called TIC TAC Primary Care Centre. This operates at lunchtimes on the school site and offers drop-in services and individual consultations.

In Great Yarmouth and Waveney District Health Authority, an outreach project was established in youth clubs because the health authority was not reaching a large enough number of young people. Robinson (1994) describes how 10 sites were selected, health advisers being appointed to each. The advisers, all with a specialist background, facilitated a considerable amount of health promotion work. Some advisers found their working conditions too noisy and smoky, but such adverse factors were used to advantage. Smoke analysers were taken into clubs to show the affects of smoking, and young people aware generally of smoking being unhealthy were shocked by more specific information on its effects.

Other work included health education games and quizzes, as well as group and one-to-one discussions on topics as diverse as skin care, toxic shock syndrome, diet, death and bereavement, homophobia, alcohol, and relationships and sex. Health notice boards were also set up, and demonstrations carried out, such as the use of contraceptives and how to perform breast and testicular self-examinations. An evaluation of the project found that an awareness of a wide range of issues had been raised, and young people's confidence in and knowledge of the health service appeared to have increased dramatically (Robinson, 1994).

McNulty and Turner (1999) outline a Northumberland Health Authority-funded project that ran from 1996 to 1998 in which young people acted as researchers to evaluate the provision of young people's sessions outside conventional health settings. They aimed to examine professional practice from a young person's perspective and to involve young people in discussions on health service development. The researchers found that the key ingredient in success of young people's health sessions was the involvement of youth workers (McNulty and Turner, 1999).

Government targets

Youth service engages in activities that address the government's identified health targets (DoH, 1992, 1999), even though these strategies fail to mention the potential of youth work. For example, 42nd Street, a project in Manchester (Sprigge, 1999), works specifically on issues of mental health, stress, breakdown and suicide in young people, particularly those from ethnic minority backgrounds, mentioned in the *Young People 2000* report as an example of good practice. The project has to date promoted a greater understanding and awareness of mental health issues, helped young people to develop coping mechanisms and created links with specialist mental health provision; it has also developed innovative work with young men that facilitates talking about emotional problems. A project in Wiltshire developed The Game as a resource for young men, also to help them to talk (Critchlow, 1998). It should be remembered that suicide is the leading cause of death in young men (DoH, 1999).

The government's target for reducing cigarette smoking among the under-16s is a cut in the present figure by 50 per cent (DoH, 1999). So far, government initiatives and advertising campaigns would seem to have had little influence on young people's smoking patterns: more sophisticated methods of influencing teenagers and young people need to be found to tackle the sense of rebellion, maturity and sophistication felt by young smokers. Youth service approaches can include work surrounding self-image and peer group pressure and conformity, and the effects of smoking on health and fitness, rather than anti-smoking rhetoric. In Rotherham, the High Energy Health initiative views smoking through a more general approach to fitness and well-being using smoke analysers, dance and exercise, as well as discussion to explore issues of smoking and health and fitness, particularly with young women.

White (1998) believes that smoking is an issue with workers who resist the authoritarian approach to working with young people that a ban on smoking implies. Many youth projects are designated smoke free either by the local council or by the young people themselves. Youth workers have provided information, encouraged discussion and facilitated young people's consideration of the issues. In these circumstances, smoking has very often been limited or banned altogether, showing that when given responsibility and autonomy, many young people will act with maturity (White, 1998).

Information and advice

The National Youth Association's Information Shops for young people, of which there are 50 spread throughout the country, offer drop-in information and advice on a wide range of topics from benefits to contraception, as well as a computer database (Beebee, 2000a). In Barking, the Association's high street shop offers music, a drinks machine and a bright, relaxing atmosphere where youth workers and other agencies can respond to local need (Beebee, 2000a). In Derby, a multi-agency partnership involved young people in the design of the drop-in centre, called The Space, with specialist clinics, and in the recruitment of staff (Chambers, 1998). In the field of drugs education, youth services have been behind many innovative projects. Good-quality youth work might be one of the most effective means of providing education advice and support to young people who are experimenting with drugs. In research carried out in Liverpool, young people did not view teachers and schools as appropriate support but mentioned detached youth workers (Young and Jones, 1996).

In Gloucestershire, there is The Info Buzz (*UK Youth*, 2000), run by the county-wide youth organisation Young Gloucestershire, which is a mobile project using a variety of methods such as quizzes, games and computer software to explore issues surrounding drugs, including alcohol and tobacco. Other projects, such as the Bristol Drugs Project, with its Fusions initiative, have gone into night clubs to offer information to young people. Web sites have recently been set up by youth projects to offer direct advice to young people; these include, for example, the Young, Queer and Safe Web site, created by the Maypole Lesbian and Gay Youth Group, and Health Initiatives for Youth UK (www.hify-uk.com). Youth organisations such as Red Cross Youth or the junior branch of the St John Ambulance Brigade offer training for young people as well as youth workers. The Red Cross recently produced a booklet on asthma aimed at youth workers (Beebee, 2000b).

Peer education initiatives

Peer relationships can assume a dominant position during adolescence, peer education being recognised as an important strategy in working with young people (Wheal, 1998). Walker (1997) describes how young people learn about sex from talking to each other; it is therefore important that the information shared is correct. The youth service has long recognised and exploited this informal method of education in group settings, in young leader and helper schemes, and in more formalised situations where young people receive specific training and support and then share their knowledge with other young people.

There are many youth service projects in which groups of young people are working with their peers on health-related issues (Cruttwell, 1999). In Redditch, for example, a young mothers group leads sessions in local schools on the realities of teenage pregnancy. Funded by Worcester Youth Service, the project uses peer education and videos to get its message across. In Sunderland, a peer education partnership targeted six youth centres to form a committed team of educators who made a video and devised training sessions on drug education (Sherriff, 1997). The Youth Link Wales peer education group produced a magazine for parents on drug-related issues. In Edinburgh, a voluntary organisation called Fast Forward, sponsored by health boards, produced a training manual for youth workers on alcohol issues.

The Health Development Agency is funding a Health in Clubs project based in 10 clubs throughout the country and managed by Youth Clubs UK, a national voluntary youth organisation. Young people are recruited and trained using a specially developed peer education framework, after which they are encouraged and supported to establish and run various local learning peer groups by themselves. Most, although not all, are focused on sexual health issues, one group concentrating on the sexual health needs of gay young men, another looking at the needs of young women.

The BREAD Youth Project in Bristol (BREAD, 1999) has worked with young people to train them to become peer educators in the field of sexual health. They visit schools and youth clubs, working directly with other young people. A peer drug education project in Somerset was evaluated as a highly successful means of getting information on drugs across to young people. The Cascade drug information service in Solihull, which trains peer educators to offer drug counselling, was established in 1992 and has trained 200 volunteers to work with over 10,000 young people. (For other good examples of similar initiatives, see Harker et al., 1999.)

The youth work contribution

The growth and development of health promotion as a distinct profession has in some instances reduced youth workers' inclusion of health education in the curriculum. The presence of the health education specialists has often meant youth workers deferring to these professionals and feeling deskilled and demotivated alongside them. Although youth workers may not have the specialist health education knowledge base, this can be provided at relatively short notice. Establishing relationships of trust and confidence is, on the other hand, a much lengthier process.

Many are now recognising the unique position that youth workers occupy and how, through working together with health service professionals, they can make an impact. The *Protecting Young People* report (DfEE, 2000b) gives youth service equal billing with schools in examples of good practice. The report recognises that youth workers are unique in being able to reach out to young people disaffected from more formal services and may be the only adults that young people trust, so the youth service is being urged to collaborate with health and social services and schools (DfEE, 2000b).

Most health services for young people are provided alongside those for either adults or children, neither of whose needs young people share. The 1989 Children Act (DoH, 1989) emphasises the fact that children and young people have the right to information, consultation and services. This, coupled with *The Health of the Nation* report (DoH, 1992), specifying for the first time targets for healthy young people, should have led to an improvement in young people's health services. Issues such as Clause 28, the Gillick ruling and concerns over providing explicit information to young people for fear of a moral backlash have, however, restricted the ability of professionals to provide effective sexual health education (White, 2000). Shropshire County Council, for example, withdrew funding from a gay and lesbian group that provided support and guidance for young people.

Statistics from the Netherlands show that the commonly held fear that increased sex education will lead to more teenage pregnancy is unfounded. The Dutch, who have a well-established sex education curriculum in schools, have experienced a decline in teenage pregnancy to 10 per 1000 girls aged 15–20 years.

Young people have, in various surveys, shown that they want access to good information, counsellors and specialist teachers, as well as settings in which they can discuss sexual matters openly and without fear of judgement (McNulty and Turner, 1999). Staff working with young people are convinced of the need for more and better sex education and an increased dialogue relating to feelings, relationships and the effects on the lives of young people if they are to deal with difficult and complicated information and make informed choices and potentially life-changing decisions. A survey by Hurrelmann and Losel (1990) showed that many young people are still not practising safer sex, perhaps because of youthful optimism and resilience or a blind hope that it will not happen to them.

When asked, young people request services and facilities similar to those provided in most youth clubs and projects. These include relaxed surroundings, warmth, music and sympathetic listening adults. With limited resources, much could be done cost-effectively to meet young people's needs by merely fully utilising the settings already available, with some extra resources to more fully meet the needs that young people have identified.

A low level of sport and physical activity in young people has recently become a concern. However, many young people freely spend their time in youth projects undertaking some form of physical or sporting activity such as football, table tennis or dancing. Many turned off by competitive team games participate in canoeing or climbing. So much more could be done with increased awareness on the part of workers and a recognition by others of the contribution that the youth service could make in this respect. The recently produced *Listen Up* report (Home Office, 2000), which interviewed 500 teenagers, found that the boys particularly wanted activities that gave them a buzz but took place in a controlled environment, such as go-karting, stock car racing and bungee jumping.

Youth workers recognise that many young people are bored, lacking access to leisure facilities and the money to do what they wish. This, coupled with their enthusiasm and energy for something dangerous and stimulating, can often lead them into the use of drugs. Here, good youth provision could play a part. With extra resources targeted not at the prevention of drug misuse but more positively at providing opportunities for sophisticated, challenging and enjoyable activities, which simultaneously address the need of young people for self-confidence and recognition, many might find drugs a less powerful attraction than at present.

Youth service activities are increasingly being regarded not only as possessing an inherent challenge, but also as a way of contributing to a healthy lifestyle and general well-being. Many projects now specifically explore the relationship of sport to fitness, body shape and weight. Sport in the youth work context once again benefits from participants having a free choice regarding participation, and with that comes the challenge for workers to ensure a range of physical activities that can be enjoyed by many different individuals. The measure of 30 minutes of exercise a day was recently publicised as a health benchmark. Many youth workers may well already provide for this or certainly could do so in the future with little extra effort, being easily able to accommodate anything from roller skating to mountain biking, or dancing to canoeing.

The other central aspect of youth provision is the development of friendship networks, these being of central importance to young people as they move through adolescence (Wheal, 1998). Adolescence is experienced as a time of stress by many young people, which may have a major impact on their health (Heaven, 1996), and social support networks can be an important factor in coping. The presence of supportive adults such as youth workers in their lives, and someone to turn to for advice or just to talk things over, can also be a key factor in coping with stress. Issues such as bullying are also relevant, as a Health Education Authority (1999) survey has recently highlighted (*Young People Now*, 1999).

If governments, health authorities and health Trusts are genuinely committed to seeing an improvement in primary healthcare for young people, there is much to be done. Identifying action is often very difficult, but in this case some answers are clear; what is missing is the real commitment to take the question seriously enough. This is not to suggest that the youth service can or should become fundamentally a health education service. However, its contribution to the health education of young people should be recognised by managers and workers within both the health service and the youth service alike, as well as by funders and others outside the service. As the examples in this chapter and many other initiatives throughout the country show, there is a great deal of good work being done that can be built on in the future for the improved health of young people.

References

Beebee, S. (2000a) Positive thinking. *Young People Now*, **131**: 13.
Beebee, S. (2000b) Asthma information. *Young People Now*, **129**: 16.
Bloxham, S. (1998) The distinctive contribution of youth and community work to the promotion of young people's sexual health. *Youth and Policy*, **61**: 173.

BREAD (1999) Annual Report available from BREAD Youth Project, 20–22 Hepburn Road, St Pauls, Bristol BS2 8UD.

Cabinet Office (1998) *Tackling Drugs to Build a Better Britain: The Government's 10-Year Strategy for Tackling Drug Misuse.* London: HMSO.

Chambers, C. (1998) A new space age. *Young People Now*, **113**.

Critchlow, J. (1998) Freedom of speech. *Young People Now*, **113**: 175.

Cruttwell, A. (1999) Sex appeals. *Young People Now*, **125**: 19–21.

Department for Education (1995) Statistical bulletin. *Young People's Participation in the Youth Service.* London: HMSO.

Department for Education and Employment (2000a) *Connexions.* London: HMSO.

Department for Education and Employment (2000b) *Protecting Young People: Good Practice in Schools and the Youth Service.* London: HMSO.

Department of Health (1989) *Childrens Act.* London: HMSO.

Department of Health (1992) *The Health of the Nation.* London: HMSO.

Department of Health (1999) *Saving Lives: Our Healthier Nation.* London: HMSO.

Harker, P., Platt, L. and Crutwell, A. (1999) *Local Action for Health.* Leicester: Youth Work Press.

Health Education Authority (1999) *Bullying as a Health Issue.* London: Health Education Authority.

Heaven, P. (1996) *Adolescent Health.* London: Routledge.

Home Office (2000) *Listen Up.* London: HMSO.

Hurrelmann, K. and Losel, M. (eds) (1990) *Health Hazards in Adolescence.* Berlin: Walter de Gruyter.

Jeffs, T. and Smith, M. (1996) *Informal Education.* Derby: Education Now Books.

McNulty, A. and Turner, G. (1999) *Report on Northumberland Young Peoples Project.* Ashington: Northumberland Health Authority.

National Youth Agency (2000) *National Occupational Standards for Youth Work.* www.nya.org.uk

New Opportunities Fund (1999) *Healthy Living Centres, Information for Applicants.* www.nof.org.uk

Policy Action Team 12. *Young People 2000.* London: HMSO.

Robinson, K. (1994) *Report on Outreach Work Undertaken in Youth Clubs by a Team of Health Advisors.* Great Yarmouth: Great Yarmouth and Waveney Health Authority.

Sherriff, T. (1997) Knowing the score. *Young People Now*, **97**: 32–3.

Social Exclusion Unit (1999) *Teenage Pregnancy.* Report. London: HMSO.

Sprigge, S. (1999) Male order. *Young People Now*, **117**: 20–1.

UK Youth (2000) (100 Summer): 8.

Walker, B.M. (1997) You learn it from your mates, don't you? *Youth and Policy*, **57**.

Warnock, P. (1999) Keeping it simple. *Young People Now*, **119**: 14–15.

Wheal, A. (1998) *Adolescence.* Lyme Regis: Russell House Publishing.

White, P. (1998) Smoke screen. *Young People Now*, **108**: 30–1.

White, P. (2000) The rise and fall of Section 28. *Young People Now*, **131**: 14.

Young, L. and Jones, R. (1996) Youth workers as drug educators. *Young People Now*, **84**: 30–1.

Young, K. (1999) *The Art of Youth Work.* Lyme Regis: Russell House Publishing.

Young People Now (1999) No. 121, 13 May.

PART V

THE VOLUNTARY SECTOR

INTRODUCED AND EDITED BY ANGELA SCRIVEN

The voluntary sector has historically played an important part in delivering the gamut of approaches and activities that we now regard as being health promoting. The two chapters that comprise this section have different functions. In the first chapter, Anderson presents a detailed overview and evaluation of the voluntary sector's contribution to health promotion. In the second chapter, Myers and Marsden revise their contribution to the 1996 edition of the book, by re-assessing the health-promoting role of self-help groups.

There are numerous key issues and debates, that emerge from both chapters. Anderson points to the amorphous nature of voluntary groups and organisations, as well as the problems associated with both defining and categorising the diversity of activity. The diffuse nature of the voluntary sector's contribution to health promotion also makes it difficult to quantify and ultimately give it the recognition it deserves. Nonetheless, it is clear from Anderson's chapter that voluntary groups and organisations make a significant contribution to meeting public health targets. Many of the goals of voluntary work embrace the ideals of health promotion, such as empowerment and advocacy, and by their very nature their work often requires and is ultimately enhanced by partnership arrangements.

There are, however, a number of dilemmas emerging from the overview. Voluntary organisations have normally been established as a direct outcome of the expressed needs of the clients they serve. They have more freedom than the statutory sector and can often act as a pressure group to bring about change. This freedom comes with a penalty. Although these organisations are often free from the shackles of normative needs and professional remits, they are frequently constrained by funding pressures, an issue that Anderson deals with in some depth. One contentious view is that voluntary organisations are often seen as plugging the gap left by inadequate statutory services; indeed, some voluntary organisations may have emerged because of the demand created by insufficient or non-existent provision available through the health and social services. Anderson makes a counterclaim by arguing that these organisations offer a different type of service, which is in many cases true, and that statutory funding might inhibit organisational freedom to act as a neutral advocate for clients. Nonetheless, it is important to recognise that the voluntary sector augments the inadequate provision of other types of health-promoting services.

Myers and Marsden, in assessing the role of self-help groups in contributing to health promotion, discuss the notion of 'joined-up thinking' and action, emphasising the aspiration for seamless services offered at the point of enquiry. They stress, therefore, the importance of the voluntary organisations and groups working collaboratively with the statutory organisations rather than offering a wholly independent service. The examples given in the chapter indicate that self-help groups are proactive in recognising both the advantages of seamless services and the scope for promoting partnership working. Notwithstanding, such partnerships should remain alert to the power relationships and the potential for imbalance in the relationships between professionals and the lay person who might be working for the voluntary organisation.

Overall, the two chapters in this section offer much to stimulate discussion and debate on the role of voluntary groups and organisations in the promotion of health within the framework of the new public health agenda.

CHAPTER 16

The Voluntary Sector and its Contribution to Health Promotion

YVONNE ANDERSON

This chapter focuses on the various ways in which voluntary agencies may contribute to the health promotion field. The term 'voluntary sector' here includes pressure groups, service providers, information services and community and self-help groups. The nature of the voluntary sector is presented as highly diverse, influencing the scope and type of health promotion and set within the context of government policy. Issues of funding are also highlighted.

Perri 6 (1991) distinguishes between the narrow voluntary sector, which includes voluntary organisations and charities, and the broad voluntary sector, which also incorporates non-profit-making organisations such as trade unions, political parties, sports clubs and trade associations. In describing the contribution to health promotion, the emphasis of this chapter will be on the narrow voluntary sector.

The diversity of the voluntary sector

The most striking feature of the voluntary sector is perhaps its great diversity. It ranges from one unpaid person working from a living room to a multi-million pound organisation employing highly professional, salaried staff. While the workplace, the school and the community have a tangible location, the voluntary sector is more amorphous and therefore more difficult to define. The Association of Voluntary Service Organisations (AVSO, 2000) describes voluntary organisations as working for the common good, with common features that include the absence of a profit-making motive, a lack of compulsion by the state and motivation arising from personal engagement. Similarly, Knight (1993) summarises voluntary work as a form of energy stemming from free will, having moral purpose and being undertaken in a spirit of independence.

The nature of the voluntary sector varies according to many factors such as geographical scope. Voluntary relief agencies, for example, provide the most essential prerequisites of health, sanitation, water and food supplies to developing countries. This is health promotion at its most fundamental level. Organisations working at a local, regional or national level in the UK make an entirely different kind of contribution.

The diversity of the voluntary sector is also reflected in the hugely different level of income generated. The Charity Commission (2000) records that 159,424 charities were registered with them in March 2000. Together, these organisations account for an annual revenue of approximately £19 billion, but within this the differential is staggering: about three-quarters of charities have an annual income of £10,000 or less, accounting for only 2 per cent of the total recorded income. This of course demonstrates that a very small number of charities are, in comparison, extremely rich.

There are obvious advantages in a voluntary organisation becoming wealthy, such as the scope for a wide influence, the ability to work alongside statutory agencies as equal contributors, the potential for attracting well-qualified staff and making a significant contribution to research and development. Disadvantages may include the inevitable bureaucracy that evolves with the growth of organisations into complex structures. Certain organisations become so large that it is difficult to differentiate them from the statutory sector in their operating methods. This might be said of the larger cancer charities, for example. Can, indeed, these large organisations remain true to their original aims and values?

In smaller organisations, the workers, usually volunteers, stay close to the client group and to the issues and problems. Although this is clearly advantageous and seems to embrace the *raison d'être* of such groups, there is a potential limitation in that people have often been motivated to start or join a group because of their personal experience of a problem. This may lead to an over-identification with clients and perhaps a particularly subjective agenda.

Smaller organisations, on the other hand, might lack the infrastructure to develop and expand the scope of their work. Many of these may not be able to afford paid staff and might even struggle to help with expenses for unpaid employees, thus denying those less financially well endowed the opportunity to act as volunteers. Small voluntary agencies may also lack the funding and organisation to support volunteers through training and development. Yet despite such difficulties, small organisations account for a large proportion of the voluntary sector and, by being small and close to the issues, offer unique services in areas that the statutory sector cannot and may not even aspire to reach.

In terms of sheer numbers alone, the voluntary sector makes an invaluable contribution to the field of health and social welfare. Estimates vary of the size of the voluntary sector in the UK. Despite the difficulty of obtaining statistics on very small local groups and those not registered as charities, the National Council for Voluntary Organisations claims that the voluntary sector employs approximately 485,000 paid workers and 3 million volunteers (NCVO, 2000).

The context of reform

Ever-increasing demands and a longer life expectancy have led to greater healthcare needs, which are difficult to meet within the resources of the National Health Service (NHS). In addition, there have been changes within the NHS that have focused on both health promotion and the inclusion of voluntary services. Enactments by government over the past two decades have led to a programme of change and reform within both the NHS and social services. The first was the introduction of the purchaser–provider system, or contract culture, within the NHS in the 1980s. Also during this time, the White Paper *Promoting Better Health* (DoH, 1987) was published, which encouraged general practitioners, through cash incentives, to run health promotion clinics and health checks. Health promotion was described as lifestyle education, behaviour change, screening and immunisation.

The *Health of the Nation* (DoH, 1992) provided for the first time a national focus for health, targeting disease reduction in key areas. Many of the objectives were identified as being achievable through an improvement in medical and healthcare, but others involved health promotion, albeit in a limited way. One way in which targets were to be achieved was by greater cooperation and collaboration between agencies, thus avoiding duplication and maximising resources. *Working Together for Better Health* (DoH, 1993) promoted the development of healthy alliances and devoted a section to working with voluntary groups. Such groups can be very important to alliances through their knowledge, commitment and ability to harness local volunteers and other resources.

Thus, both health promotion and the voluntary sector were placed on the national agenda. Partnership continued to be a theme of the new Labour government, which published its White Paper, *The New NHS: Modern, Dependable* in its first year of office (DoH, 1997). The key theme of this document was the 'third way', which meant keeping what had worked and discarding what had failed.

The third way in this instance referred to 'a system based on partnership and driven by performance' (DoH, 1997: 10). This was the leitmotif of the rationale for New Labour and was echoed in the naming of voluntary and community organisations as 'The Third Sector' (Home Office, 1998). Emanating from *The New NHS* has been the establishment of Health Action Zones and the Commission for Health Improvement. Both programmes are being led strategically by health authorities and involve joint planning groups that embrace all the relevant statutory and voluntary organisations in a local area or district.

In 1998, the government, in partnership with the voluntary sector, published *The Compact*, an agreement to shape future working together. Following its publication, the formation of action plans has begun in areas of strategy, policy and practical implementation. The voluntary sector could not

be better placed amidst this agenda of reform and modernisation to implement the principles of social inclusion, participation and citizenship:

> The work of voluntary and community organisations is central to the Govern-
> ment's mission to make this the Giving Age. They enable individuals to contribute
> to the development of their own communities. By so doing, they promote citizen-
> ship, help to re-establish a sense of community and make a crucial contribution to
> our shared aim of a just and inclusive society. (Home Office, 1998: 3)

The scope for health promotion

Voluntary organisations have a variety of purposes; some have a single function, but others, more usually, have two or more. A primary function of many
voluntary organisations is to act as *service providers*. A major service provider
is the hospice movement, perhaps an unlikely candidate for health promotion
as it is concerned with the care of terminally ill people, but the very emphasis
on the quality of life remaining, including the aims of dignity, respect and
freedom from pain, is an example of health promotion at a tertiary level. The
hospice movement, which also embraces Marie Curie Cancer Care and
Macmillan Cancer Relief, has introduced new perspectives on the way in
which terminally ill people are cared for. Providing pioneering research and
development in symptom control and pain relief, the movement has had a
profound influence on mainstream medicine. It is disappointing that such
advances could not have been made within the NHS and that carers and
patients have to rely on a voluntary organisation for something as fundamental as palliative care. It is also important to remember that voluntary
organisations do not simply plug a gap left unfilled by the statutory services.
The voluntary sector is predicated both on morally committed action and
specialist focus.

Another function of voluntary organisations is to act as *pressure groups*,
attempting to promote change in large statutory bodies such as the NHS.
There are long-standing groups, such as MENCAP and ad hoc groups, which
campaign for a single, short-term aim, such as to save a local hospital from
closure. They may be extremely effective at mobilising public opinion, which
in turn puts pressure on policy makers to change their plans. A major difficulty for the voluntary sector in this field, as in others, is that it cannot
compete with larger organisations, whether public or private, so minority
causes or less popular, less media-friendly concerns become lost.

Many voluntary organisations have a role in *education and information*,
replying to letters, using the media, organising courses or producing
newsletters and magazines. Contributions may be made to editorials in
women's magazines, and advice can be given on specific health matters
occurring in soap operas for radio and television. There are also telephone
advice lines providing information on a wide range of topics. The children's

charity Childline produces factsheets, all encompassing information from young people themselves, on a range of health-related topics including bereavement, bullying, child abuse, suicide and eating problems. The strength of a service such as this is that the information is appropriately marketed to its target group, using members of the group to participate in the developments. Here can be found a good example of the contrast between the voluntary and statutory sectors. The former is organised around a specific group and particular issues for that group, while the latter is organised to meet the much more global and generalised needs of a heterogeneous population.

Other functions can include *community development*, as, for example, with residents' associations, social clubs and playgroups. Some of these, such as well woman groups, have a health promotion topic as their central focus, whereas health issues are covered more indirectly in others. A neighbourhood group, with very limited resources, will normally work on a client-centred basis, dealing with issues as they arise. The concerns of clients often have a health-related impact, as, for example, with preventing dogs fouling the pavements, or campaigning for traffic-calming measures.

In the culture of evidence-based practice, the extent and effectiveness of health promotion within the voluntary sector demand to be assessed. As stated in *The Compact*:

> Voluntary and community organisations make a major and incalculable contribution to the development of society. (Home Office, 1998: 6)

'Incalculable' is more than just political rhetoric. The contribution to health promotion made by the voluntary sector can arguably never be measured, for several reasons, the most salient perhaps being that many people helped by voluntary organisations are themselves powerless and disenfranchised. These are the people without a voice – literally in the case of the 4,590,000 contacts made to Samaritans in 1999, of which 38 per cent were silent. An aim of successive administrations in the NHS has been to reduce the number of suicides and attempted suicides. It is highly debatable that people with suicidal feelings are articulate and motivated enough at that point to negotiate help from the statutory services.

Health promotion may exist indirectly within organisations where the stated purpose does not offer an explicit clue to its presence. This is amply illustrated in the case of Victim Support. The stated purpose of this organisation is to help and support the victims of crime; it does not hold a specific remit for health promotion. Much of the work of Victim Support volunteers, however, has clear potential for promoting health, in helping people to cope with traumatic events, serious losses and dangerous life-change events that, left alone, could cause long-term mental health problems (Murray-Parkes, 1993).

Whatever the predominant function(s) of a particular voluntary organisation, there is a central linking theme, that of *empowerment*. It has been suggested (Rissel, 1994: 40) that 'There are few concepts in health promotion with as much potential as that termed "empowerment". It embodies the *raison d'être* of health promotion.' The concept of empowerment, embraced by health promotion, has its origins firmly rooted in the social action and community participation ideals, which are the underpinning philosophies of the modern voluntary movement. Furthermore, volunteering may be seen as health promoting in itself.

The foregoing discussion has centred upon organisations and groups, but individuals also contribute, as the following extract demonstrates:

> Volunteers contribute to the NHS and Social Care in a range of ways: for example, driving patients to and from appointments, collecting prescriptions, translation for non English speaking patients, running hospital shops and tea shops. There are also opportunities for befriending, helping disabled people and those with mental illness to lead a normal life, helping at parent and toddler groups, entertainment and the arts, visiting patients in hospital and the community, or by fundraising for special projects. The NHS also relies on volunteers for blood, tissue and organ donation. (DoH, 2000: 1)

Constraints posed by funding

Voluntary organisations may be funded in a number of ways, many receiving core funding from the statutory agencies, although some of the larger charities rely almost solely on voluntary contributions and fund raising. An example of the latter is the major cancer charities, some of which operate on multi-million pound budgets. Voluntary organisations are increasingly looking to the commercial world for funding and resourcing in other ways, and therein lies a dilemma. The voluntary sector relies on public faith as well as public donations. In a recent report, 70 per cent of people questioned agreed that one of the most important aspects of a charity was the set of values it represented. The two factors most closely associated with voluntary organisations were that they are caring and non-profit based (NCVO, 2000). Once an organisation becomes very large, or starts to rely upon the statutory sector for funding, its core values can come under fire.

Insecure funding for many voluntary organisations can make long-term planning difficult. Short-term funding means that posts may only be offered on a time-limited contract, making it difficult to attract staff. Additionally, some small organisations have a quite simple structure, often relying on one key individual, which can create difficulties if that person leaves. Problems with staffing and funding can clearly lead to a lack of consistency and continuity.

Funders have a right to be involved, through policy and procedure, in how their resources have been used by the organisation, those bodies represented on the management committee normally achieving this. Other members of that committee would be representatives of other community groups, staff and volunteers. Management committees can be a dynamic example of collaboration in action, but there is also the potential for conflict when the members represent different interest groups. Fund-raising committees are also a feature of many organisations; their duties range from organising sophisticated national campaigns to instigating local charity events.

Whatever the scale of a fund-raising activity, it is always made easier when the clients are seen as deserving or are made to look appealing. Public consciousness is raised by marketing campaigns that range from publicity material accompanying door-to-door collections through to huge media events such as a telethon and Live Aid. The debate for the voluntary sector is whether such campaigns are morally defensible or are exploitative and contradictory to the core aims and values of the organisation. It is of course an easy task to portray children and cancer sufferers as a worthy cause, but some groups, including immigrants, refugees and other minorities, do not have this advantage. Whither the health promotion for them?

To summarise, the voluntary sector is large and diverse, voluntary services arising out of morally committed action. The multi-functional nature of voluntary groups determines the scope for health promotion. Both health promotion and the voluntary sector have been placed on the government agenda. There are shared values and philosophies between the two and most health promotion taking place in the voluntary sector is indirect, implicit or unseen, lying within broad defining principles. Finally, issues arising from funding methods cause concern for the scope of smaller organisations and also raise ethical questions for the larger ones.

In conclusion, the participative nature of voluntary services is in keeping with the more empowering models of health promotion, those which are client centred, ecologically driven and focused on social change and community development. The very act of volunteering may be health promoting in itself.

This chapter has embraced the paradox that the contribution of the voluntary sector to health promotion, although almost certainly immense, is so diffuse and broadly defined, that it cannot be quantified. The overall contribution of the voluntary sector to the promotion of health is effectively summed up by the following, which acts as an apposite final testimony to the work of voluntary organisations:

> [Voluntary services] act as pathfinders for the involvement of users in the design and delivery of services and often act as advocates for those who otherwise have no voice. In doing so they provide both equality and diversity. They help to alleviate poverty, improve quality of life and involve the socially excluded. (Home Office, 1998: 6)

References

Association of Voluntary Service Organisations (2000) *What Voluntary Service is All About.* http://www.avso.org/volunteerdef.html

Charity Commission (2000) http://www.charity-commission.gov.uk

Department of Health (1987) *Promoting Better Health.* London: HMSO.

Department of Health (1992) *The Health of the Nation.* London: HMSO.

Department of Health (1993) *Working Together for Better Health.* London: HMSO.

Department of Health (1997) *The New NHS: Modern, Dependable.* London: HMSO.

Department of Health (2000) *Volunteering in Social Care.* http://www.doh.gov.uk/volunteering/index.htm

Home Office (1998) *The Compact on Relations between Government and the Voluntary and Community Sector in England.* http://www.homeoffice.gov.uk/vcu/compact.pdf

Knight, B. (1993) *Voluntary Action.* London: Centris.

Murray-Parkes, C. (1993) Bereavement as a psychosocial transition: process of adaptation to change. In Stroebe, M.S., Stroebe, W. and Hanssor, R.O. (eds) *Handbook of Bereavement.* Cambridge: Cambridge University Press.

National Council for Voluntary Organisations (2000) http://www.ncvo-vol.org.uk

Perri 6 (1991) *What is a Voluntary Organisation? Defining the Voluntary and Nonprofit Sectors.* London: NCVO Publications.

Rissel, C. (1994) Empowerment: the holy grail of health promotion? *Health Promotion International,* 9(1): 39–47.

CHAPTER 17

A Self-help Approach to Health Promotion

JAN MYERS AND KATE MARSDEN

In the intervening five years since the first edition of this book, there have been considerable changes affecting the development of health and social care provision, which have impacted on national and local voluntary organisations. These changes have included a host of government Green and White Papers (see, for example, DoH, 1999a, b), strategies for modernising national health services and local authorities, a move to primary care settings for health improvement and local sensitivity to assessing needs, alongside the special initiatives such as Health Action Zones to speed up the processes of addressing inequalities.

A central feature in all of these new initiatives is the place of the patient, service user and carer in measuring and demonstrating how effective our health and social services are in making a difference to people's health and well-being. This greater recognition of the patient's voice, along with issues of practice development, quality services and outcomes in giving best value to the end customer, means that patients groups and self-help groups are becoming increasingly recognised as a valuable source of consumer feedback. In the context of developing Primary Care Trusts, the regeneration of communities and lifelong learning, this chapter looks at the important role that self-help and mutual aid can play for individuals and the increased need to develop meaningful relationships across sectors in relation to partnership working, patient participation and active health promotion.

The connection between self-help and health promotion

From the outside looking in, the voluntary sector can be a confusing array of interest groups, diverse communities and different organisational structures. Their size and complexity ranges from that of large international organisations, such as aid agencies, to that of smaller national and local registered charities, and through to more informal groups such as self-help and mutual support groups. The legal status, policy framework and accountability of this range of organisations and groups will vary depending on a number of factors. These include charity registration, registration as a company, whether

189

the organisation has paid employees, whether there are service-level agreements or funding agreements in place, the amount of money a group fund-
raises or holds and the aims, objectives and membership criteria.

Self-help groups fall towards one end of the continuum. Many arise spon-
taneously to meet local need or in response to gaps in services, are informal,
often hold meetings in people's homes and in many ways fall outside many
of the formalised monitoring procedures set up by statutory agencies. At the
same time, they provide, and are increasingly recognised as providing, a vital
support role to individuals in need, to people learning to live with long-term
medical conditions and to marginalised communities. As Mullender and
Ward (1991: 12) explain:

> in groups personal troubles can be translated into common concerns. The demor-
> alising isolation of private misfortune... can be placed in the course of collective
> enterprise with a new sense of self-confidence and potency, as well as tangible prac-
> tical gains which individuals on their own could not contemplate.

However, mutual aid also begins with 'the desire to take oneself in hand'
(St Armand and Clavette, 1992: 18). In this way, in order to become a
member of a self-help group, an individual must be conducive to, or seeking,
change. For example, persons who join Alcoholics Anonymous (AA) do so in
the knowledge that they are alcoholic and want to do something about it.
Here, the people themselves define the *problem* (being alcoholic) and determine part of the *solution* (joining and participating in AA). In this way, if we
take Thorogood's suggestion in Bunton and MacDonald (1992: 77–80) that
health promotion should 'start where people are developmentally... start
where people are emotionally... start where people are socially', self-help
groups can provide a good thermometer for all three areas.

Moreover, both health promotion and self-help are concerned with a
holistic picture of the person. This wide approach to health promotion is
defined by the World Health Organization, quoted in Fieldgrass (1992: 7),
where health promotion is seen as a 'unifying concept for those who recognise the need for change in the ways and conditions of living, in order to
promote health'. A key element of this is 'supporting the principle of self-
help and self-care movements to allow people to form their own directions
for managing the health of their own community' (Fieldgrass, 1992: 8). This
process of enabling people to increase control over, and to improve, their
health (WHO, 1986) then provides a guide to an essential and effective link
between health professionals and self-help groups.

Defining self-help

Toffler (1981) has looked at the rapid growth of self-help and with it the
basic shift in roles of what he terms 'prosumers', that is, people relying on

themselves for things for which they have previously depended on others. With this comes the confluent change of the professional expert to 'listener, teacher and guide who works with the patient or client' (Toffler, 1981: 279). Groups may educate their members not only in disease management, but also in the healthcare system and the way it works.

The evaluation of such activities often features research into professionally led therapy or support groups, so it is important to be aware of the general defining characteristics of self-help groups. A self-help group is a group of people who come together around a common problem, condition or concern. This usually involves people who are directly affected, such as those with multiple sclerosis and/or their carers or the partner of a person with dementia. Many self-help groups are disease related, but the diversity of groups covers issues such as bereavement, sexual abuse, gender issues, drug and alcohol misuse, eating disorders, parents groups and mental health issues. The consistent factor is that they are run by and for their members. For a full definition of a self-help group, visit Self Help Nottingham's Web site (see References).

Linking self-help and the promotion of healthy living

With the increasing emphasis on inclusive ways of working to promote and encourage healthy living, self-help groups can be seen to have a role in the primary and secondary prevention of ill health. There are many examples of this in areas such as reducing the number of crisis admissions to hospital or encouraging positive attitudes to diet and exercise after cardiac rehabilitation. This role is increasingly being supported by research into the effectiveness of self-help and mutual aid activities.

Kurtz (1988), cited in Kyrouz and Humphreys (2000), found that, out of 129 members of a group for people with manic depression and depression, 82 per cent reported that they were coping better after they joined a self-help group. In addition, the percentage of people being admitted to psychiatric hospital before joining was 82 per cent, whereas 33 per cent reported hospital admission after involvement in the group. The longer the period of membership and the more actively people were involved in the group, the more they said that their coping had improved. Similarly, Emrick et al. (1993) looked at the experience of AA members. They found that the longer a person had been a member, coupled with an increase in participation and responsibility over time, for example leading a meeting or sponsoring other members, the more that member stayed sober.

The level of participation and leadership is a significant factor in enabling people to feel more in control of their health, in gaining increased knowledge, in opening up options and choices, and on increasing commitment both to themselves and to other members. Wilson and Myers (1998) give the example of Rose, a carer. Through group involvement, Rose started to take part in health and social services consultation meetings and planning services for carers. She began to be asked to give talks to professionals about her experiences and, aged 70, went back to college to take a course in presentation skills. In order continuously to learn, develop and change, people have to participate, and the greater the participation in the group, the more individuals gain (Reissman, 1965). de Ridder et al. (1997) would also see this in terms of moving from an emotional response to coping to a more problem-solving stance, which they consider to be more effective in the long term in adapting to and coping with enduring health problems.

How health professionals support self-help initiatives can also affect the success or failure of a group. This can be a simple act such as displaying a group's poster. On the other end of the scale, it may be help with material resources, putting people in touch with the group, access to meeting rooms or support and training for group members to enhance their skills in running a group.

Health promoters can also act as a signpost to other services when professional back-up is needed. The strength of this help is that it is sensitive background support, based on community work, enabling principles and being offered over a long period (Wilson, 1994). It also recognises and values the experiential knowledge of group members and the mutual benefit that this relationship can have for group and professional alike.

Linking health promotion with other health and welfare policies

Fosse and Roeiseland (1999) examine Norwegian health promotion policy and highlight the growing relevance of health promotion and public health matters to other fields of policy and decision making. In the UK, we can see similarities in relation to the growing emphasis on local authorities' responsibility and influence on health, the move towards pooled budgets and shared healthcare planning and provision.

This move towards 'joined-up thinking' and action emphasises the promotion of seamless services offered at the point of enquiry. Self-help groups involved in a series of network meetings, organised by one of the authors, to discuss health improvement in coronary heart disease and stroke, gave examples of several incidents concerned with the development of prescriptions for exercise. They pointed to the need for this initiative to be tied into town planning (pavements often not being in a condition to provide stable walking conditions for a person with one side affected by stroke, or the ill-thought-out placement of lowered kerbs at crossings), leisure facilities and staffing (equipment often being available at swimming pools to help people in and out of the water but staff not always being trained to use it), transport policies and access issues. Here, we can see the insight of patients recovering from heart attacks or living with disability caused through stroke in translating theory into practice. It also underlines the value of involving patients, service users and carers at all levels of service planning, provision and evaluation in determining cost-effective and appropriate services.

Jason et al., cited in Kyrouz and Humphreys (2000), studied how self-help can be useful in the workplace. Two smoking cessation programmes were run at 43 companies, involving over 400 participants. Approximately half the participants watched a television programme and were given a self-help manual to help quit smoking. The second group also had six self-help support meetings. The initial rate of quitting smoking in the companies that used self-help groups was significantly higher (41 per cent) than that of the companies that did not (21 per cent). Of those smoking, group members smoked fewer cigarettes per day, with a lower nicotine and tar content. After three months, of those taking part in self-help groups, 22 per cent had continued not to smoke, compared with 12 per cent in those companies with no self-help group.

The value of self-help activities and peer support is also shown by Pisani et al. (cited in Kyrouz and Humphreys, 2000) in sustaining behavioural change after a specific health intervention. Here, it was found, in a study of over a hundred alcoholic patients admitted for short-term treatment, that attendance at AA meetings following discharge improved abstinence more than did adherence to prescribed medication.

Promoting active alliances

For some professionals, the lack of professional expertise in a group may raise concerns about the benefits and risks associated with self-directed groups. Marmar et al., cited in Kyrouz and Humphreys (2000), studied the difference between a controlled trial of brief therapy and self-help for women bereaved after the death of their husbands. The authors basically found that self-help groups worked just as well as therapy and that symptoms of stress and depression were equally reported, as were improvements in coping with home and work.

There is often a need to examine power relationships between professionals and lay people. A closer collaboration can lead to greater familiarity between groups and professionals, and issues such as these can be discussed more openly. Ashworth et al. (1992: 1431) make the observation that 'the effort to treat patients and clients as genuine participants, in fact as genuine human beings, ought to be axiomatic to a profession widely understood to have human interpersonal relationships at heart'.

Ashworth et al. (1992: 1434) also state that the 'use of jargon by professionals ensures that the client remains an outsider, unable to participate fully with the expert group'. This is supported by St Armand and Clavette (1992: 111), who give an example of the information-giving and intermediary role that self-help groups have for newly diagnosed patients: 'Dr X will tell him things that he doesn't understand, and I'll explain it in simpler terms instead of big fancy words.'

Holman and Lorig (2000: 526) state that, in dealing with chronic diseases in which the aim is to enhance quality of life, 'the key to effective management is understanding the different trends in illness patterns and their pace'. Often 'doctors cannot accurately detect the trends themselves. The patient knows them better, and provides information and preferences that are complementary to the doctor's professional knowledge' (Holman and Lorig, 2000: 526). This is where self-help group members become experts on their own condition.

Where an emphasis is put on patient-centred care and individualised care packages, McEwan, cited by Cahill (1996: 563), asserts that patient participation 'is widely recognised as a good thing as it results in increased patient responsibility and a commitment to health and health-promoting behaviours'. While the stress has been placed on links with patients and service users through self-help groups, there has been a steady growth in the number of groups for carers over the past 10 years. The government paper on *Modernising Social Services* (DoH, 1998) used the General Household Survey of Great Britain 1995 and noted 5.7 million carers, 1.7 million providing care for 20 or more hours a week. Improving quality of life and keeping people healthy also need to be carer focused. If individuals feel disempowered in their relationships with professionals, self-help groups can often offer a collective voice to raise issues, mediate or act in an advocacy role.

Patient participation: a central role in health promotion

Cahill (1996: 563) also asserts, that 'according to Meyer (1993) patient participation is a major thread of health promotion'. This can be either on an individual, one-to-one, basis or a group, one-to-many, basis. A locally based cardiac support group actively promotes health at its monthly meetings by inviting a wide variety of speakers, ranging from cardiac specialists, paramedics, physiotherapists and pharmacists, to social welfare professionals, who can advise on employment, benefits and aids. Here, the health promotion professionals take an active role in supporting the group by attending meetings when asked to by the members. The running, and therefore control and management, of the group is the responsibility of the members. One local group, Positive Health, finds that links with professionals help to create a better understanding of health and of the way in which health agencies work. The group has a generalist approach to health and invites speakers on a wide range of subjects, their rationale being that group members may at some point in their own life be affected by, for example, a stroke, dementia or osteoporosis. In this way, there is awareness raising, a positive approach to growing old and an active way of providing space to relax and learn. This also raises confidence in the health services, an important issue in health promotion.

Another development from self-help organisations (such as Arthritis Care and the Manic Depression Fellowship, national organisations with small, more local branches and support groups), one following on from the North American trend, is the growth of self-management programmes. In these, self-help group members have been trained in self-management techniques, the continuous use of medication, pain management, coping with life changes and anticipating and interpreting change as the disease progresses. Kate Lorig, Professor of Medicine at Stanford University School of Medicine, has been a major contributor to this field, particularly in terms of chronic arthritis, and states, 'an important element for participants is learning from each other, and the principal reason for benefit is growth in confidence in their ability to cope with their disease' (Holman and Lorig, 2000: 527). The benefits of mutual support and reciprocity are again emphasised, providing an opportunity for developing partnership working and dialogue between self-managers and health professionals.

Looking to the future

The growth of communication technology and the speed at which some self-help groups, particularly in North America, have utilised this to set up on-line groups expands the opportunities for involvement and inclusion. Traditionally seen as relating to groups for older people of 35 years and over, particularly women, the Internet provides space and opportunities for targeting younger males and other hard to reach populations. With the increasing development of mobile communications and, on the horizon, digital television and communications technology, the ability to access information and networks globally is increasing, which presents new challenges and opportunities. At a pan-European level, there are health promotion projects such as Eurolink Age, a not-for-profit network of organisations and individuals working on good practice and policy related to ageing. They advocate local community-led action in influencing public policy decisions as having the additional benefit of empowering individuals, groups and communities (Walters, 1998).

A community-centred approach can move decision making closer to people at the grass-roots level and resonates with democratic ideals and the concepts of civil society and social capital. The belief is that better local communities will provide better lives for people and empower them to make health-promoting choices about their lives and their lifestyles (Fosse and Roeiseland 1991). In this way, self-help groups can be seen as a convenient setting in which to implement new healthy living approaches. It has always, however, to be recognised that groups have their own agenda and needs. Some groups may not always be conducive to healthy living approaches or organised in a way that can facilitate such approaches. Efforts to encourage this may only serve to divert the group and resources away from their original aims and objectives of supporting their members.

The role of self-help in health promotion is about providing an opportunity to speak to others in similar situations, to provide information and raise awareness, and to enhance quality of life, personal growth and development. It is about taking control and recognising an ability to respond to the situation in which a person may find him or herself.

Perhaps a final word can be left to the practitioners of the future. The project described involved setting up an Internet home page for health promotion using a broad community approach to health. Men's and women's health issues were included, as were details of community health projects being undertaken by the Monash University Medical School and a detailed listing of health resources, including self-help groups in the area (Victoria, Australia):

> The third year students who designed this site believe strongly that self-help groups will play an increasingly significant role in the maximisation of health in the future. (Gradstein et al., 1996)

References

Ashworth, P.D., Longmate, N.A. and Morrison, P. (1992) Patient participation: its meaning and significance in the context of caring. *Journal of Advanced Nursing*, 17: 1430–9.

Bunton, R. and MacDonald, G. (1992) Health promotion discipline or disciplines. In Bunton, R. and MacDonald, G. (eds), *Health Promotion: Disciplines and Diversity*. London: Routledge.

Cahill, J. (1996) Patient participation: a concept analysis. *Journal of Advanced Nursing*, 24: 561–71.

Department of Health (1998) *Modernising Social Services*, Chapter 1: Adult services: independency, consistency and meeting people's needs. URL: http://www.doh.gov.uk/dhhme.htm

Department of Health (1999a) *Saving Lives: Our Healthier Nation*. London: Stationery Office.

Department of Health (1999b) *Reducing Inequalities: an Action Report*. London: Stationery Office.

de Ridder, D., Depla, M., Severens, P. and Malsch, M. (1997) Beliefs on coping with illness: a consumer's perspective. *Social Science Medicine*, 44(5): 553–9.

Emrick, C.D., Tonigan, J.S., Montgomery, H. and Little, L. (1993) Alcoholics Anonymous: what is currently known? In McCrady, B.S. and Millar, W.R. *Research on Alcoholics Anonymous: Opportunities and Alternatives*. New Brunswick, NJ: Rutger Centre for Alcohol Studies, pp. 41–75.

Fieldgrass, J. (1992) *Partnerships in Health: Collaboration between the Statutory and Voluntary Sectors*. London: HEA.

Fosse, E. and Roeiseland, A. (1991) From vision to reality? The Ottawa Charter in Norwegian health policy. *Internet Journal of Health Promotion*. URL: http://www.ijhp.organisation/articles/1999/1

Gradstein, D., Hofman, S. and Reuben, Y. (1996) Health Promotion on the Internet. *Internet Journal of Health Promotion*. URL: http://www.ijhp.organisation/articles/1996/1

Holman, H. and Lorig, K. (2000) Patients as partners in managing chronic disease. *British Medical Journal*, 320: 256–7.

Kurtz, L.F. (1988) Mutual aid for affective disorders: the Manic Depressive and Depressive Association. *American Journal of Orthopsychiatry*, 58(1): 152–5. Cited in Kyrouz, E.M. and Humphreys, K. (eds) *A Review of Research on the Effectiveness of Self-Help Mutual Aid Groups*. URL: http//www.mentalhelp.net/articles/selfres.htm

Kyrouz, E.M. and Humphreys, K. (2000) *A Review of Research on the Effectiveness of Self-Help Mutual Aid Groups*. URL: http//www.mentalhelp.net/articles/selfres.htm

Meyer, J. (1993) Lay participation in care: a challenge for multi-disciplinary teamwork. *Journal of Interprofessional Care*, 7(1): 57–66.

Mullender, A. and Ward, D. (1991) *Self Directed Groupwork*. London: Whiting & Birch.

Reissman, F. (1965) The helper therapy principle. *Journal of Social Work* 10(2): 27–32.

St Armand, N. and Clavette, H. (1992) *Self Help and Mental Health: Beyond Psychiatry*. Canada: Canadian Council on Social Development.

Toffler, A. (1981) *The Third Wave*. London: Pan.

Walters, R. (1998) Promoting the health of older people – making it happen. *Internet Journal of Health Promotion*. URL: http://www.ijhp.organisation/articles/1998/1

Wilson, J. (1994) *Social Care Research 60: Self Help Groups and Professionals*. York: Joseph Rowntree Foundation.

Wilson, J. and Myers, J. (1998) *Self Help Groups: Getting Started, Keeping Going*. Nottingham: RAW.

World Health Organization (1986) *Ottawa Charter for Health Promotion*. Ottawa: WHO.

Web sites:

American Self Help Clearing House on-line: http://www.mentalhelp.net/selfhelp
Institute for Health Promotion Research, Toronto: http://www.ihpr.ubc.ca
Long Term Medical Conditions Alliance: http://www.lmca.demon.co.uk
Monash Health Promotion Project, Australia: http://www.monash.edu.au/health
Self Help Nottingham: http://www.selfhelp.organisation.uk
UK Government sites: http://www.doh.gov.uk/dhhome.htm

PART VI

WORKPLACE

INTRODUCED AND EDITED BY JUDY ORME

The workplace has increasingly been recognised as an important setting in which to consider health issues. Work in itself can be seen as contributing to public health and as causing ill health in many ways. The breadth of this complexity demands its visibility in order to ensure that a range of appropriate health promotion and health protection policies are developed at different levels.

The chapters that follow between them contribute to this visibility. The dilemmas presented by the current provision of workplace health promotion and occupational health services are debated. The context of growing flexible employment patterns and the impact on health in terms of insecurity and risk are highlighted. The chapters collectively uncover the strengths and weaknesses of the workplace as a setting for achieving public health targets and emphasise the importance of developing multi-agency collaboration in workplace health promotion.

Norma Daykin analyses why the workplace does not provide a neutral environment for health promotion activity. The visibility of the social, economic and political factors that shape the working environment is central to the appropriate development of workplace health strategies.

Tom Mellish examines the role of trade unions in promoting health. The original chapter in the first edition, written by Sarah Veale and Marc Beishon, has been through a major update to ensure that the impact and implications of the recent policy initiatives are analysed. As Mellish highlights, one of the primary roles of trade unions has always been to ensure that employees are working in safe and healthy conditions, and the principles underpinning the achievement of this are discussed. One important aspect discussed at length in the chapter is access to occupational health services. Mellish details a realistic analysis of the dilemmas posed by the existing provision and illustrates his argument with some excellent examples of national and international initiatives.

The final chapter in this section, written by Jennifer Lisle, highlights a number of key areas central to the role of the occupational health services in promoting health. These include first the need for the provision of a safe and healthy workplace, second, the importance of employees being able to contribute effectively to the organisation's goals and enhance their own personal well-being, and third, the need to promote the optimal physical, mental and emotional health of all employees.

International comparisons demonstrate the inconsistency of the provision of occupational health services first between countries and second between organisations of different sizes within countries. Very recent policy focusing on occupational health services is discussed, and the opportunities provided by this new strategic approach are analysed.

The complementary nature of the chapters in this section does help to tease out the complexities involved in health promotion in this challenging setting. The dilemmas produced by the social, economic and political context of workplace health are critically analysed, making an important contribution to current public health debates.

CHAPTER 18

Overview of Health Promotion in the Workplace

NORMA DAYKIN

Strategies for promoting health at work can take place at many different levels. In its broadest sense, workplace health promotion is concerned with the prevention of ill health and the promotion of positive health and lifestyle among people in the workplace. The workplace does not, however, provide a completely neutral environment for health promotion activity. Work is itself recognised as contributing to health and causing ill health in many ways. Furthermore, the social, economic and political factors that shape the working environment mean that workplace health promotion represents a complex challenge.

This complexity is illustrated by the fact that a wide number of agencies, each with different goals and purposes, could legitimately be involved in promoting health at work. These include statutory bodies charged with the regulation of health and safety at work, occupational health services provided by employers, trade unions, National Health Service (NHS) health promotion services and voluntary organisations. Furthermore, within the workplace itself, health can be affected positively or negatively through a wide range of activities, for example organised activity in response to legislative health and safety requirements, routine management practices and communications styles, trade union campaigns for an improvement in working conditions and single-issue health promotion campaigns on, for instance, smoking or healthy eating. Effective health promotion in the workplace therefore relies on developing collaboration and communication between a wide range of agencies and individuals.

The effects of work on health

The effects of work on health can be positive as well as negative. In general, employees seem to fare better than the unemployed across a range of mortality and morbidity indicators (DoH, 1999). Work can, however, also be harmful to health, directly through occupational injury, disease and psychological stress, as well as indirectly (Harvey, 1988). The indirect effects of work on health are of particular relevance to the debate about the appropriateness of workplace health promotion. These include behavioural responses to stress such as smoking and alcohol consumption, as well as the indirect consequences of work that fails to provide insufficient income to sustain health. Relatively little is known, however, about these broader effects of work on health. While there are statutory requirements for the reporting of occupational accidents and certain diseases, a number of difficulties have served to limit research in this area. As a consequence, the reported levels of work-related disease and ill health represent the 'tip of the iceberg' (Levy and Wegman, 1995: 9). One of the difficulties affecting research in this area stems from the dominance of the medical model. The discourse of Western scientific medicine, with its emphasis on the doctrine of specific aetiology, in which every disease is understood in relation to a single cause, has strongly influenced our understanding of the relationship between work and health. This doctrine is reflected in conventional definitions of occupational disease. These restrict the definition to particular conditions in relation to which specific causative factors in the workplace can be clearly identified, measured and controlled (WHO, 1985).

This definition excludes many conditions, such as those which do not originate at work but are partially caused or exacerbated by adverse working conditions. Also excluded from view is the way in which the risks of work-related ill health interact with personal and social characteristics such as class, ethnicity and gender, reinforcing established inequalities. Furthermore, this narrow definition overlooks conditions that may be compounded by personal behaviours such as smoking or alcohol consumption. In response to these limitations, the World Health Organization has advocated a broader definition of work-related ill health, which recognises the complex and multi-causal nature of many problems. This broader definition provides a sounder basis for the development of workplace health promotion activities than that provided by conventional definitions of occupational disease.

A further difficulty in the development of knowledge about workplace health issues is the lack of methodological sensitivity that has characterised research in this field (Harrison, 1996; Doyal, 1998; Messing, 1998, 1999). Epidemiological bias has limited the understanding of health and work issues for particular groups. In relation to gender, most knowledge about general health issues in the work environment has been based on the male employment experience. The use of the term 'work' itself reflects this problem. This term is most commonly used to refer to paid employment outside the home. Women are, however, often involved in work activities that are broader than this (Doyal, 1995, 1999; Lloyd, 1999; Payne, 1999). These include unpaid domestic work and childcare as well as informal or unregulated employment such as that in the sex industry. People engaged in these activities have health promotion needs that may mirror those of conventional employees, yet little is known about these needs. It may be necessary for workplace health promotion campaigns to target a wider range of activities than those suggested by conventional notions of 'work'.

Changing conditions of work and their implications for workplace health promotion

Recent global trends, including the increased mobility of capital and sectoral shifts in investment and employment from manufacturing to service industries, have influenced the experience of employment in a number of ways, features of the UK experience being summarised by Church and Wyman (1997). Overall, the economic activity rate has risen for some groups and declined for others. Hence the women's economic activity rate has continued to rise over the past few decades, while among men, it has fallen. As well as being related to the decline in manufacturing employment and the growth in unemployment, this pattern has been reinforced by other trends, such as a rise in early retirement. In the late 1990s, just over half of all men aged 60–64 were economically active compared with 80 per cent in 1971. The rising economic participation rate among women is particularly apparent for some groups, including mothers (although single parents are less likely than married and co-habiting mothers to be employed). In addition to the growth in service sector employment, in which women are strongly represented, there is a trend of an increase in part-time and flexible working. Women are six times more likely than men to be in part-time employment.

This pattern has a number of implications for health (Daykin and Doyal, 1999). First, there may in the future be a decline in traditional forms of occupational disease, such as pneumoconiosis among miners. However, the long period between exposure and the onset of such conditions means that any decline will not reveal itself for many years. Furthermore, globalisation means that many occupational risks, such as those relating to asbestos, are simply transferred from developed countries to poor countries, where regulatory frameworks are undeveloped (Johanning et al., 1994).

Women's rising participation in the labour force will undoubtedly result in their increased exposure to many kinds of occupational health risk. At the same time, their continued responsibility for childcare and domestic work means that issues of health and work for women will arise from multiple roles and exposure patterns. Just as gender-sensitive research strategies are needed to understand these issues, so gender-sensitive health promotion strategies will be needed to address them and promote positive health for women at work.

Changing working conditions may also have a material effect on the organisation of work, making workplace health initiatives difficult to sustain. Privatisation, contracting out and self-employment, for example, can often lead to the loss of, or reduced access to, traditional occupational health services provided by employers. Health promotion activities are unlikely to thrive in such settings. Similarly, the growth of small firms may affect the provision of occupational health and health promotion. Research suggests that workers and managers in small companies perceive issues of health and risk differently from those in large companies, and that such employers are less likely to view themselves as having a legitimate reason to interfere in the private domain of employees' health (Eakin and MacEachen, 1998).

Changes in working conditions, such as the introduction of new technology, are likely to necessitate new health promotion strategies as new groups of workers become exposed to existing problems. This can be seen in the case of musculo-skeletal disorders, which have traditionally affected workers in manufacturing industry but increasingly affect other groups such as journalists and teachers (Watterson, 1999). The growth in flexible, often insecure, employment may also affect the pattern of risk. Insecurity has been linked to ill health at an individual and population level (Wilkinson, 1996). Just as researchers will need to pay increased attention to the psychosocial aspects of work and risk in the future, those providing workplace health promotion may need to take issues of stress and insecurity as their starting point.

The focus and impact of workplace health promotion

Research suggests that most worksite health promotion initiatives reflect a rather narrower set of concerns than those outlined above. Furthermore, there is little evidence of effective multiprofessional working in this field. Worksite health promotion initiatives have historically been more strongly developed in the USA than in other countries. This is partly because US employers' responsibilities in relation to employees' health insurance create a stronger incentive to offer preventive health programmes. During the 1980s and 90s, programmes developed in a number of areas ranging from smoking, alcohol and drug education, to weight control, exercise, stress management and screening for cancer and cardiovascular risks (Hollander and Lengermann, 1988; Lovato and Green, 1990). UK and other European employers gradually became aware of the perceived benefits of health promotion initiatives, including reduced costs, reduced sickness absence and improved morale (Wynne, 1992).

Workplace health promotion has, however, tended to be concentrated in large, public sector organisations with trade union representation (HEA, 1993; Sanders, 1993; Daykin and Cockshott, 1996). These organisations are also more likely to provide occupational health services to their employees, meaning that workplace health promotion may serve as a useful extension to these services but that workers who do not have access to such services may be doubly disadvantaged.

This leads us to consider the characteristics of workplace health promotions services in terms of their focus and impact. During the 1980s, the individualistic focus of much health promotion activity was strongly criticised

(Naidoo, 1986). This focus was seen as being particularly problematic in relation to the workplace, where the sensitivity to notions of risk, responsibility and blame is heightened. The relatively narrow focus on lifestyle and behaviour has been presented as at worst insulting and at best irrelevant to workers who are every day faced with hazards that stem from poor work organisation and harmful processes (Watterson, 1986). In this context, even such strategies as hazard education carry the danger of transferring the responsibility for health protection from employers to employees.

While caution is needed in adopting simplistic lifestyle approaches within the workplace, we have seen that current economic trends render the experience of work and employment increasingly complex. It is not always possible to identify a clear-cut distinction between 'lifestyle' and 'workplace' health issues. This is because, for many people, the boundaries between work and leisure or domestic life are becoming increasingly blurred. Furthermore, the aetiology of many conditions is complex, with work risk spilling over into other spheres. For example, stress at work may influence health-related behaviour such as smoking and alcohol consumption. This may partly explain the observed association between conditions such as liver cirrhosis and lung cancer and the membership of particular occupational groups (Leigh and Jiang, 1993; Kjarheim and Andersen, 1994). This calls for a rethinking of the relationship between health and work, which may itself lead to a reformulation of the debate about workplace health promotion over the decades. In the future, work-related health problems are likely to demand flexible, multi-disciplinary prevention strategies. These need, however, to be based on an acknowledgement and understanding of the ways in which work contexts, processes and relationships can affect health and well-being.

As this debate has continued, it has proved difficult in practice to broaden the focus of workplace health promotion. A recent review of the Health at Work in the NHS initiative reported that few organisations can demonstrate a long-term, proactive and sustained approach to improving the quality of working life (HEA, 1999). This report demonstrated that workplace health initiatives tend to be narrowly conceived, the strongest motivating factor being compliance with legislative requirements rather than the desire to promote positive health. While employers increasingly offer services such as counselling for employees, strategies for addressing the health impact of organisational and management problems are less in evidence. Furthermore, the access to such services remains patchy, and they are often viewed suspiciously by staff, who fear that they may not be sufficiently confidential. This reinforces findings from qualitative case study research in both public and private sector organisations (Daykin, 1998), as well as accounts from specialist practitioners in the field (Pickvance, 1999).

This brings us to consider the impact of workplace health promotion. One area of debate has been that of the impact of workplace health promotion on established health inequality. Health activity in the workplace may in two ways reinforce the 'inverse care law' (Tudor Hart, 1971), whereby those in greatest need enjoy less access to healthcare and receive poorer services. First is the issue of access to health promotion in the workplace. The organisation of paid employment means that relatively disadvantaged groups, such as low-paid workers and minority ethnic groups, tend to be concentrated in unreg-ulated private sector employment where the risks are high and workplace health initiatives are little in evidence (Phizacklea and Wolkowitz, 1995; McBarnette, 1996). In addition, within organisations, many facilities that may impact on employees' health take the form of perks for relatively senior staff. Hence in one study, company cars and private medical insurance were five times more likely to be provided than childcare facilities and three times more likely to be provided than paternity leave (Daykin and Cockshott, 1996). Needless to say, these benefits were available only to a small minority of relatively well-paid staff.

Linked to this issue of access to health benefits is the issue of the take-up of workplace health promotion. Evidence suggests that even when workplace health initiatives are open to all staff, the take-up rate is higher in certain groups. In fact, the groups least likely to participate in workplace health promotion activity are those groups who experience the poorest general health as well as at the greatest risk of occupational ill health and injury (Daykin, 1998). The characteristics of workers more likely to participate in health promotion activity include white collar salaried employment and a relatively high level of education (Alexy, 1991; Sanders, 1993; Stonecipher and Hyner, 1993).

Promoting health at work

Recent policy initiatives have recognised the importance of the workplace as a site for health promotion. In *Saving Lives: Our Healthier Nation* (DoH, 1999), the workplace is highlighted as representing both problems and opportunities. The document notes the scale of work-related ill health, 2 million people suffering from a work-related illness and a consequent 20 million working days being lost in Britain in 1995. Particular attention is given to the problems of psychosocial stress, with an estimated 5 million working days lost each year from stress, depression or anxiety. The link between an improvement in the workplace and reducing health inequality is also established in the document. It suggests that stress at work is a key factor contributing to the disease burden disproportionately affecting those in lower socio-economic groups. Hence reducing stress at work is seen as an important element contributing to the attainment of public health targets in relation to coronary heart disease, stroke and mental health.

If these targets are to be achieved, a change in the focus of workplace health promotion is needed, as are efforts to make health promotion acces-sible and relevant to relatively disadvantaged groups. This means overcoming a number of barriers that have impeded the development of health promotion in the workplace in its broadest sense. These barriers arise from the socio-political context in which debates and strategies for health at work have emerged.

The development of the statutory and legislative framework for the regulation of employment and the provision of occupational health and health promotion services have historically been influenced by power relationships within wider society. One perspective suggests that this has been to the detriment of workers, who may remain rightly suspicious of workplace health initiatives. It has been argued that theory and practice relating to health and work have often served the interests of employers at the expense of those of workers (Navarro and Berman, 1981; Sass, 1996). Hence the status accorded to 'scientific' knowledge has been seen as justifying exploitative and dangerous methods and processes of production. Furthermore, occupational health professionals have been viewed as lessening the attention paid to work hazards, minimising the scale of occupational disease or denying its work relatedness, and seeking to explain health problems with reference to workers' own habits and behaviour (Weindling, 1985; Watterson, 1986). Whether or not this perspective can be endorsed, it is apparent that the occupational health services have been dominated by employers' management and personnel requirements rather than being focused on prevention and rehabilitation in relation to work-related ill health. This creates a potential ethical minefield for workplace health promoters, who must work sensitively and consensually in a context in which the balance of power and resources may be uneven.

This discussion highlights the need for an improvement in three areas. First, strategies are needed to empower relatively disadvantaged groups of workers to themselves identify and address health needs in the workplace. Participatory research has been advocated as one means of empowerment (Loewenson et al., 1999). Participatory research builds upon lay epidemiology and involves workers in identifying, investigating and proposing solutions to workplace health issues. The balance of knowledge and resources is, however, often skewed against these groups. Thus, in order to strengthen workplace health promotion, it is clear that sources of information and support that are independent of employers are needed.

The NHS's specialist health promotion services may have an important role to play in this area. These services are, however, often limited and lack extensive knowledge and experience of workplace issues. Furthermore, they are not underpinned by any statutory obligation on the part of the NHS to provide occupational health and health promotion services to the general population. If workplace health initiatives are to be meaningful to low-paid and disadvantaged workers, they are likely to start by addressing employees' concerns about the work environment. Primary care professionals are the group who are most likely to encounter such concerns, but these groups also lack both specialist knowledge and the impetus of statutory obligation in this area.

This highlights a second area in which improvement is needed in the form of the provision of specialist independent information and advice to support workplace health promotion. One source of such information could be the specialist occupational health services that currently exist in some countries. In Denmark, for example, employers contribute to a collective service that provides information and instigates action in the workplace on behalf of employers and employees alike (Pickvance, 1996). In the UK, there are a number of innovative services, such as the Sheffield Occupational Health Project, which provides independent, multi-disciplinary expertise and support to both employees and employers. The project is based within primary care, where the majority of workplace health problems are first presented (Pickvance, 1999). The extent of such services is, however, currently limited, and, in addition, these services remain reactive and not backed by statutory powers. Nor do they currently have the resources to extend into the field of health promotion.

This highlights the third area in which improvement is needed: that of multi-agency collaboration. Workplace health promotion has many different meanings, but the definition that supports the implementation of current public health targets is wide and includes a number of elements including risk management, disease surveillance and management, occupational health provision, organisational change, counselling and lifestyle health promotion. The different agencies charged with these functions need to work together to respond to established and emerging health needs of the workforce.

References

Alexy, B.B. (1991) Factors associated with participation and non participation in a workplace wellness centre. *Research in Nursing and Health*, **14**: 33–40.

Church, J. and Wyman, S. (1997) A review of recent social and economic trends. In Drever, F. and Whitehead, M. (eds) *Health Inequalities. Decennial Supplement*, Office for National Statistics, Series DS No. 15. London: Stationery Office.

Daykin, N. (1998) Workplace health promotion: benefit or burden to low paid workers. *Critical Public Health*, **8**(2): 153–66.

Daykin, N. and Cockshott, Z. (1996) *Workplace Health Promotion and Low Paid Employment. Report of Research in the Bristol Area*. UWE/Bristol Area Specialist Health Promotion Service.

Daykin, N. and Doyal, L. (eds) (1999) *Health and Work: Critical Perspectives*. London: Macmillan.

Department of Health (1999) *Saving Lives: Our Healthier Nation*. London: Stationery Office.

Doyal, L. (1995) *What Makes Women Sick? Gender and the Political Economy of Health*. London: Macmillan.

Doyal, L. (1998) Introduction: women and health services. In Doyal, L. (ed.) *Women and Health Services. An Agenda for Change*. Buckingham: Open University Press.

Doyal, L. (1999) Women and domestic labour: setting a research agenda. In Daykin, N. and Doyal, L. (eds) *Health and Work: Critical Perspectives*. London: Macmillan.

Eakin, J.M. and MacEachen, M. (1998) Health and the social relations of work: a study of the health-related experiences of employees in small workplaces. *Sociology of Health and Illness*, **20**(6): 896–914.

Harrison, B. (1996) *Not only the 'Dangerous Trades'. Women's Work and Health in Britain 1880–1914.* London: Taylor & Francis.

Harvey, S. (1988) *Just an Occupational Hazard? Policies for Health at Work.* London: King's Fund Institute.

Health Education Authority (1993) *Health Promotion in the Workplace.* London: HEA.

Health Education Authority (1999) *Developing and Sustaining Workplace Health in the NHS.* London: HEA.

Hollander, R.B. and Lengermann, J.J. (1988) Corporate characteristics and worksite health promotion programmes: survey findings from Fortune 500 companies. *Social Science and Medicine*, **26**: 491–501.

Johanning, E., Goldberg, M. and Kim, R. (1994) Asbestos hazard evaluation in South Korean Textile Production. *International Journal of Health Services*, **24**(1): 131–44.

Kjarheim, K. and Andersen, A. (1994) Cancer incidence among waitresses in Norway. *Cancer Causes Control*, **5**: 31–6.

Leigh, J.P. and Jiang, W.Y. (1993) Liver cirrhosis deaths within occupation and industries in the California Mortality Study. *Addiction*, **88**: 767–79.

Levy, B.S. and Wegman, D.H. (1995) Occupational health in the global context: an American perspective. In Levy, B.S. and Wegman, D.H. (eds) *Occupational Health: Recognising and Preventing Work Related Disease.* London: Little, Brown.

Lloyd, L. (1999) The wellbeing of carers: an occupational health concern. In Daykin, N. and Doyal, L. (eds) *Health and Work: Critical Perspectives.* London: Macmillan.

Loewenson, R., Laurell, A.C. and Hogstedt, C. (1999) Participatory approaches in occupational health research. In Daykin, N. and Doyal, L. (eds) *Health and Work: Critical Perspectives.* London: Macmillan.

Lovato, C.Y. and Green, L.W. (1990) Maintaining employee participation in workplace health promotion programs. *Health Education Quarterly*, **17**(1): 73–88.

McBarnette, L.S. (1996) African-American women. In Bayne-Smith, M. (ed.) *Race, Gender and Health.* London: Sage.

Messing, K. (1998) *One Eyed Science: Occupational Health and Women Workers.* Philadelphia: Temple University Press.

Messing, K. (1999) Tracking the invisible: scientific indicators of the health hazards in women's work. In Daykin, N. and Doyal, L. (eds) *Health and Work: Critical Perspectives.* London: Macmillan.

Naidoo, J. (1986) Limits to individualism. In Rodmell, S. and Watt, A. (eds) *The Politics of Health Education.* London: RKP.

Navarro, V. and Berman, D.M. (1981) *Health and Work under Capitalism: An International Persepective.* New York: Baywood.

Payne, S. (1999) Paid and unpaid work in mental health: towards a new perspective. In Daykin, N. and Doyal, L. (eds) *Health and Work: Critical Perspectives.* London: Macmillan.

Phizacklea, A. and Wolkowitz, C. (1995) *Homeworking Women: Gender, Racism and Class at Work.* London: Sage.

Pickvance, S. (1996) Towards multidisciplinary prevention services. *Occupational Health Review*, (Sep/Oct): 27–32.

Pickvance, S. (1999) Occupational health issues and strategies: a view from primary health care. In Daykin, N. and Doyal, L. (eds) *Health and Work: Critical Perspectives*. London: Macmillan.

Sanders, D. (1993) *Workplace Health Promotion: A Review of the Literature*. Oxford: Oxford Regional Health Authority.

Sass, R. (1996) A strategic response to the occupational health establishment. *International Journal of Health Services*, 26(2): 355–70.

Stonecipher, L.J. and Hyner, G.C. (1993) Health practices before and after worksite health screening. *Journal of Occupational Medicine*, 35(3): 297–306.

Tudor Hart, J. (1971) The inverse care law. *Lancet*, 1: 4005–12.

Watterson, A. (1986) Occupational health and illness: the politics of hazards education. In Rodmell, S. and Watt, A. (eds) *The Politics of Health Education*. London: RKP.

Watterson, A. (1999) Why we still have 'old' epidemics and 'endemics' in occupational health: policy and practice failures and some possible aolutions. In Daykin, N. and Doyal, L. (eds) *Health and Work: Critical Perspectives*. London: Macmillan.

Weindling, P. (ed.) (1985) *The Social History of Occupational Health*. London: Croom Helm.

Wilkinson, R. (1996) *Unhealthy Societies*. London: Routledge.

World Health Organization (1985) *Identification and Control of Work Related Diseases*. Technical Report No. 174. Geneva: WHO.

Wynne, R. (1992) *Innovative Workplace Actions for Health: An Overview of the Situation in Seven EC countries*. Dublin: European Foundation for the Improvement in Living and Working Conditions.

CHAPTER 19

Trade Unions and Health Promotion

TOM MELLISH

In recent years, trade unions have become important agents in helping to initiate and sustain workplace health promotion. During the 1980s and 90s, many unions developed their traditional health and safety functions to cover pressing workplace health issues such as work-related upper limb disorders and stress, as well as cooperating with employers in broader campaigns such as cancer screening, healthier eating and initiatives to cut the consumption of tobacco, alcohol and drugs (HEA, 1992).

It is important to recognise that one of the primary roles of trade unions has always been to ensure that employees are working in safe and healthy conditions (TUC, 1992). Unions, however, see this role as part of a democratic process of collective bargaining rather than as a direct appeal to interfere with the rights and choices of an individual. Unions concentrate on socio-economic factors that can be negotiated with employers and not on lifestyle issues.

Acknowledging this distinction is crucial to gaining the cooperation of unions in workplace healthy alliances. However, with the long-standing concern for industrial health and safety issues, unions have begun to adopt the view that it is inconsistent to separate certain health issues from the more traditional shop-floor emphasis on safety. The Trades Union Congress (TUC) has always maintained that the two are inseparable. It would be inconsistent for example, to provide healthy eating options in the staff canteen if workers were then expected to return to a shop floor with a dangerously high noise level. Some so-called health promotion initiatives are viewed with great suspicion by unions (TUC, 1992). There have been some thinly veiled attempts to weed out less healthy employees for redundancy, but in a context of full consultation, and a consistent health and safety policy across an organisation, unions are not likely to be hostile to health promotion activities.

Background to trade unions

Today in Britain there are 73 trade unions affiliated to the TUC, representing nearly 7 million members (TUC, 1999b). There are trade union members in every industry and service, including top managers, scientists, teachers, printers, skilled workers, labourers, radiographers, musicians and airline pilots.

Part-time workers are increasing as a proportion of trade unionists in employment, and the current union density, that is, the number of workers in unions, is overall about 30 per cent of the total workforce (DfEE, 1999). Unions are organised in different ways, depending on their size and the type of employee they represent. A large union, such as the GMB, has a national office with departments covering different services and trade groups, as well as a number of regional offices staffed by full-time officials. A small union such as the Union of Textile Workers has no regional offices (TUC, 1999b).

Most unions also have a large number of lay officers, those not employed by the union but undertaking certain duties in the workplace, such as health and safety representatives. In total, there are about 2000 full-time union officers, the majority of whom work for the large unions. There are more than 200,000 lay safety representatives in Britain, and more than 70 per cent of working people have access to one of these volunteer officials (TUC, 1999b).

Since the Health and Safety at Work Act 1974, safety representatives have become an integral part of the management of health and safety in the workplace. They have the right to investigate accidents, inspect the workplace and be consulted by an employer about health and safety training programmes and the introduction of new production methods or machinery into the workplace. Inspectors from the Health and Safety Executive (HSE) also talk to union safety representatives when carrying out their inspections and may discuss their findings with them. The TUC trains more than 7,000 safety representatives each year in setting up effective health and safety committees. A number of larger unions have a health and safety committee made up of national executive members.

More than 218 people die each year in workplace accidents (HSE, 2000). There are just under 29,000 major injuries and an estimated 10,000 deaths as a result of work-related health damage, as well as 4,000 arising from asbestos-related diseases. The HSE *Self-reported Work-related Illness Survey* (HSE, 1998) revealed that 1.3 million people who had worked in the past year suffered from work-related ill health. As a result of those injuries, a total of 24.3 million working days were lost and over 27,000 people were forced to give up work. The HSE estimates that the cost to British industry of occupational accidents and ill health is over £18 billion annually.

It is hardly surprising therefore that safety and certain direct health hazards are a priority for unions. For example, the TUC recommends that safety committees check health records on absenteeism, referrals to the occupational health department, data on biological monitoring, hearing tests, the causes of death of past employees and the results of surveys seeking out specific health problems, such as lower back pain, skin problems, respiratory complaints, work-related upper limb disorders and symptoms of stress (TUC, 1994). At a national level, health and safety has survived into the 21st century as one of the few remaining areas that is conducted on a tripartite

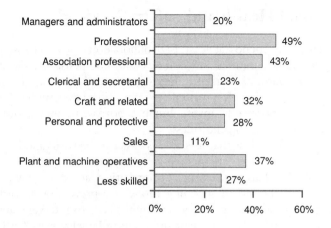
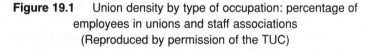

Figure 19.1 Union density by type of occupation: percentage of employees in unions and staff associations (Reproduced by permission of the TUC)

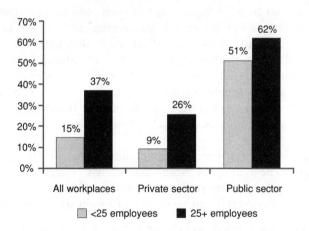
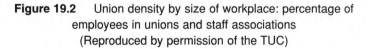

Figure 19.2 Union density by size of workplace: percentage of employees in unions and staff associations (Reproduced by permission of the TUC)

basis, government, employers and union representatives working together to develop national health and safety policies and legislation. Trade unions in other countries have similar concerns about health and safety in the workplace, with varying degrees of statutory support (European Trade Union Technical Bureau, 1989).

A National Health and Safety Dividend

Britain currently spends at least £18 billion every year on lost production, treating workplace injuries and illnesses, and compensating the victims. The balance of resources is currently heavily weighted towards clearing up after the event, which is largely a wasted resource. If the government's golden rule is that we may borrow to invest, but not borrow to spend, our health and safety system is breaking the rules.

One reason for this is that it is always easier to be wise (and bountiful) after the event, when there are people needing attention and assistance, than beforehand. But that is the essence of prevention, and if too few employers are willing to take the risk of spending money on prevention in order to avoid spending it on the victims, the government needs to intervene and prime the pump. As a result, the government should itself benefit, as well as business and workers benefiting, by reaping the rewards of lower National Health Service (NHS) expenditure, lower benefit payments and an increased tax revenue.

The TUC believes that, with adequate safeguards, existing expenditure on the outcome of poor health and safety – such as employer liability insurance, Industrial Injuries Disablement Benefit and NHS expenditure on work-related injuries and ill health – could be put to better use. Small and medium-sized enterprises should be a principal target of such redistribution (large firms to some extent carrying out just such a system internally). This is because these stand most to gain and will be most influenced by the immediacy of tax breaks and grants rather than the longer-term promise of reduced costs.

The government should create a Safety Dividend, using existing funds such as employer liability insurance, Industrial Injuries Disablement Benefit and NHS expenditure on work-related injuries and ill health, as well as raising new funds to invest in prevention and rehabilitation, with:

- a national injury and illness insurance fund based on employers' liability premiums, to be used by the Health and Safety Committee to buy insurance cover from individual insurers on the basis of standard policies including a recognition of good risk management and a right to rehabilitation;

- a safety investment bond, to increase access to occupational health services and stimulate innovation through grants for small firms and intermediaries along the lines of the Department of Health's Section 64 grants; and

- tax breaks for expenditure on rehabilitation and prevention, accessed through the Reporting of Injuries, Diseases and Dangerous Occurrences Regulations (RIDDOR) reporting and the meeting of audited safety targets.

The TUC believes that all investment in health and safety should be treated as capital investment, because it involves a long-term commitment to the human capital of the business, and should be taxed as such. This should cover preventive activity as well as rehabilitation.

A National Health and Safety Partnership

The government should create a National Health and Safety Partnership to encourage employers and unions to build on the success of safety representatives and safety committees in halving major injury rates, including:

● developing the role that safety representatives can play in promoting effective health and safety risk management, through the use of Provisional Improvement and Prohibition Notices;

● developing the role of unions in assisting small firms with risk assessment and risk management, and in representing and educating their members through roving safety representatives;

● developing the skills and qualifications of safety representatives through courses fully funded by the new National Learning and Skills Council.

The TUC believes that the involvement of the workforce is crucial to good standards of health and safety, and that health and safety systems function best when unions and employers work together. The role of safety representatives is crucial to this. As cited above, the evidence suggests that a full system of consultation with safety representatives and a joint safety committee involving unions and employers produces a major injury rate of 5.3 per thousand workers, compared with a rate of 10.9 where no consultation takes place.

Union safety representatives bring an enormous amount to any partnership. This includes the ability to benchmark what happens in their workplace with what they know from union sources about other workplaces; knowledge and skills related to health and safety provided on the basis of high-quality training provided by the TUC and unions (which produced the result that, in an HSE study of industry's perception on chemical hazards, safety representatives were more aware than their line managers); and an ability to reflect the views of the workforce, checking the reality of what managers think or suppose is happening at the sharp end. Safety representatives also play a key part in transmitting messages from management to the workforce about the advisability of compliance with safety standards, interpreting them in ways that their fellow workers will understand and adopt.

Safety representatives could, however, do a great deal more to improve safety standards in the workplace if they were given a more active role in risk management. Many unions already encourage their representatives to get involved in risk assessment (rather than just commenting on it when the risk assessment has been done), and many employers involve their safety representative in both the strategic and the day-to-day management of health and safety. Drawing on international examples, the TUC believes that this role could be strengthened if safety representatives were able to ensure their involvement in health and safety decision making. One way to achieve this is by giving safety representatives the authority to serve what are known as

Provisional Improvement or Prohibition Notices. These would have the same effect as an Inspector's Notice except that they are open to challenge by employers, who can call in an inspector if they suspect that the basis of the Provisional Notice is flawed. The TUC would accept some safeguards against abuse, such as the role of the Inspectorate, and we also accept that safety representatives would need to demonstrate competence to serve such notices before acquiring the authority to do so (see below).

The positive benefits that safety representatives bring could be extended to other workplaces. Safety representatives currently cover about a third of the workforce, mostly in larger workplaces. They are, rightly, drawn from the workforce they represent, so that they understand that workforce and have legitimacy as its representative voice. In the light of the Employment Relations Act, their influence may be extended to cover more workplaces where unions gain recognition. The TUC does not, however, believe that recognition is a requirement for safety representatives to play a positive role, and we believe that there should be a right for workers who belong to trade unions to appoint safety representatives to represent themselves, regardless of recognition rights. In one particular sector, the offshore oil sector, this would have the effect of integrating the current, unique system of representation into that in operation on the mainland under the 1977 Safety Representatives and Safety Committee Regulations.

Some workplaces, however, are simply too small for this to be a realistic prospect. Where there are only five employees, some of whom are not union members, it is not likely to be feasible to expect one of them to take on the role of a safety representative, or easy for the workplace to provide the requisite time off. The TUC's research into safety representative experiences in small firms suggests that such enterprises do not have the internal management structure on which much health and safety law is based and therefore need external support to manage many of the functions that would produce better health and safety standards. For these small firms, access to safety reps would be a major asset, delivering not only representation for the workforce, but also access to support, information and advice that would otherwise have to be paid for through consultancy fees. Although safety representatives do not have legal responsibilities in this field, and their advice could not be relied on in court, their views would, for most practical purposes, be valuable input for most small firms.

For these reasons, the TUC believes that the Swedish system of roving safety representatives ought to be adopted in the UK. Such a system does already exist in Britain under the 1977 Safety Representatives and Safety Committees Regulations. This is in the music and performing arts sector, in which the Musicians' Union and Equity, the actors' union, are entitled to appoint safety representatives for workplaces where there is no recognition and no internal safety representative, and a similar experiment has been attempted in the agricultural sector by the Transport and General Workers

Union. Two lessons arising from that experiment were that voluntary schemes of this type do not work and that legal rights are needed.

As mentioned above, safety representative training provided by the TUC and unions is of a high quality (as assessed by certification and inspection bodies). The TUC has recently agreed with the Institution of Occupational Safety and Health that acquiring credits through the TUC safety representative training system should provide access to professional safety qualifications. At the moment, however, the access to such courses is restricted, partly by the TUC and unions' ability to fund the courses and partly by the reluctance of employers to make arrangements for safety representatives to go on the courses. It is not so much that the legal entitlement to time off for training is being breached (because where it is, unions use their legal entitlements to remedy such breaches) but that too many safety representatives feel pressured into staying at work because their work will not be covered, bonuses will be jeopardised and so on.

The TUC believes that there should be a more formal recognition that safety representative training is a vital contribution to the health of the nation, individual enterprises and workforces, as well as that employers should see an involvement in union representation (as has happened in a ground-breaking agreement between Manufacturing, Science, the Finance Union and Legal & General) as part of the career path of a successful employee. This would be assisted, and levels of safety representative expertise extended, if the new National Learning and Skills Council recognised safety representative training as being worthy of full exemption from fees, rather than providing partial funding as at present.

Access to occupational health services

The TUC has welcomed the Health and Safety Commission's 10-year strategy for occupational health in Great Britain (HSC, 2000), and was involved in its drafting. This section will not, however, comment on the many good aspects of that strategy but will focus instead on one area that is not within the scope of the strategy and needs government intervention to deliver – access for everyone to an occupational health service (TUC, 1999a).

Millions of workers in smaller firms or self-employment do not have access to any occupational health advice, information or provision, and nor do the small firms themselves. The TUC believes that the government should provide access to occupational health for everyone at work through a Community Healthy Workplace Service. This would extend access to and improve the efficiency of existing provision, increase the liaison between the existing providers and plug the gaps at local level (especially for small firms and the self-employed) by putting an occupational health and safety expert in every Primary Care Group.

Previous governments have excused themselves from accusations of non-compliance with the European Union's Framework Directive by hiding behind the fig leaf of the NHS. This suggests that since everyone has access to the NHS, and since the NHS provides health services regardless of the source of the injury or illness, everyone has access to an occupational health service. Union experience has demonstrated that this is nonsense. The NHS has neither the resources nor the expertise to provide everyone with access to occupational health services. Unions in the health service regularly complain that it is not even able to provide such access for all its own staff, although there are areas of excellence in the NHS that should be built on.

The TUC does not, however, believe that there is much merit in developing an all-embracing national occupational health service on top of what existing provision there is. Many employers, often in partnership with unions, have established perfectly appropriate provision, which it would be foolish to duplicate or replace. An occupational health service that is based on the experience of a particular workplace and workforce is generally preferable to a free-floating service because it will have a focus, access to the working environment and a body of experience that cannot be reproduced externally. Our proposals on tax breaks for expenditure on health and safety would provide an incentive to expand and extend these services. There are also examples of local provision, such as Occupational Health Projects based on a multi-disciplinary team of medical and occupational specialists and overseen by representatives of the stakeholders (the local community, trade unions, employers and so on) which the TUC would want to see expanded and properly funded.

Instead of a single national service, therefore, the TUC prefers the model to provide access to legal services already advanced by the Lord Chancellor's Department – a Community Healthy Workplace Service. This would address the gaps in existing provision, such as the needs of small firms or the self-employed (as well as the unemployed), thus also helping to meet the government's aims of supporting small business and combating social exclusion.

As mentioned above, the TUC preferred model is the Occupational Health Project. The Sheffield and Liverpool projects (as well as several others around the country) have been able to develop imaginative solutions to the problems faced in their communities. The feedback generated from health services into better prevention in the workplace would probably not be possible without the involvement of employers and unions. The TUC believes that, where it can be demonstrated that the local support exists, the government should fund such projects directly out of the national injury and illness insurance fund.

That level of local support will not, however, exist everywhere, as the patchwork development of Occupational Health Projects has shown. The Community Healthy Workplace Service should therefore also ensure that occupational health services are available in other parts of the country. The TUC has been working with the Forum of Private Business over recent months to develop a framework and published a joint statement on occupational health in small firms in July 1999.

Others will need to contribute to the Community Healthy Workplace Service too. In particular, the TUC believes that the statutory Employment Medical Advisory Service within the HSE should, on top of its functions of advice and inspection in industry (necessarily limited by its small size), act as a champion for occupational health provision in each health authority area. This would ensure that each Health Improvement Plan deals appropriately with occupational health.

The TUC also believes that workers (and their safety representatives) have a role in increasing the awareness of health problems at work, for example by carrying out self-assessments of work-related health problems. One way to do this is by using the body-mapping technique, which was piloted in October 1999 by the TUC and BackCare to highlight the problems of back strain for women in the workplace.

And finally... getting back to work

There is for most people no clear distinction between prevention, compensation and rehabilitation/treatment. Only by learning the lessons of the latter can the former be effective. The TUC would like to see a system whereby people who suffer an occupational injury or illness receive fair compensation and appropriate treatment and are assisted to retain or return to work (by rehabilitation, retraining or adaptations to the workplace).

This is one area in which the UK lags behind almost every other industrial nation. In response, the TUC has been working with the insurance industry to develop a model for a new approach. The TUC believes that the government should ensure that everyone injured or made ill by work has access to a personal Back to Work Plan, involving:

- tax breaks triggered by reporting requirements under RIDDOR;
- extending the health and safety policies that employers are required to have to cover rehabilitation;
- individual case managers arranging the delivery of the Back to Work Plan;
- minimum quality standards for providers.

The starting point for rehabilitation must be the accident or illness itself: one problem with the current position in Britain is that NHS provision is triggered only by a visit to the general practitioner or by beginning the process of seeking civil compensation – both usually at far too late a stage. This will require a better reporting of injuries and illnesses than RIDDOR currently provides. The current level of reporting is far too low, at about 40 per cent (lower in some industries). One of the reasons why RIDDOR is ineffective is that it looks like bureaucratic pen pushing, filling in forms for the sake of it or so that the form filler can be punished. If RIDDOR actually triggered state subsidies or tax breaks for rehabilitation, that might make it work.

When an injury has been reported, there needs to be a mechanism in place to ensure that the sufferer enters a rehabilitation arrangement. In Australia, employers are strongly encouraged to develop a rehabilitation policy that they negotiate with their workforce. The TUC believes that this in itself will encourage a substantial increase in rehabilitation by stimulating employers to address the problem as part of the active management of sickness absence and health generally. The TUC feels that voluntary encouragement will only reach the best employers. It holds that a vehicle does exist for developing such a policy as a legal requirement without adding much to the burdens on business, that is, the written health and safety policy that all employers with five or more employees are required to have. It would be comparatively simple to require employers to include rehabilitation provision in the policy (based on guidance), and existing requirements on consultation would lead to workforce/safety representative involvement in that policy.

Having a policy does not itself mean, however, that action will be taken,. TUC investigation of the Australian system has indicated that the key to delivery is the position of a case manager to oversee the rehabilitation. This person is unlikely to be medically trained, thus avoiding the problem of a medical model of retention and rehabilitation. He or she does, however, have access to the information on rehabilitation and to the resources that are available to make sure that an employee gets a viable Back to Work Plan and that it is put into effect.

A third crucial element is that government should establish minimum quality standards for rehabilitation, whether these apply to the NHS (overcoming an apparent lack of consistency around the country) or to private providers. In addition, wherever it is sited, the provision needs to be collectively funded, which means either through taxation (the NHS) or through compulsory insurance provision, as already exists for compensation. Why do we require employers to spend money on paying injury victims but not to spend money on rehabilitating them?

References

Department for Education and Employment (1999) *Labour Force Survey*. London: HMSO.

European Trade Union Technical Bureau for Health and Safety (1989) *Prevention at the Workplace*. Belgium: New Imprimerie Duculot.

Health Education Authority (1992) *Health Promotion in the Workplace: The Trades Union Movement*. London: HEA.

Health and Safety Commission (2000) *Securing Health Together*. Sudbury: HSE Books.

Health and Safety Commission (2000) *Safety Statistics Bulletin 1999/00.* Sudbury: HSE Books.

Health and Safety Commission/Department for the Environment, Transport and the Regions (2000) *Revitalising Health and Safety.* Wetherby: DETR.

Health and Safety Executive (1998) *Self-reported Work-related Illness in 1995.* Sudbury: HSE Books.

Health and Safety Executive (2000) Statistical Report. Sudbury: HSE Books, www.hse.gov.uk/hsestats.html

Trades Union Congress (1992) *Report to 1992 Congress.* London: TUC.

Trades Union Congress (1994) *Report to 1994 Congress.* London: TUC.

Trades Union Congress (1999a) *Better Jobs for Better People.* London: TUC.

Trades Union Congress (1999b) *Report to 1999 Congress.* London: TUC.

CHAPTER 20

Organisational Health: A New Strategy for Promoting Health and Well-being

JENNIFER LISLE

The working population is a key group within society, comprising 27 million people in the UK and some 155 million in the European region. The working population is therefore a very major target group for health promotion.

Workplace health promotion has the potential to reach a large number of people but needs to be considered within the changing context of work. Throughout the 1980s and 90s, the rapid pace of change has continued to produce a great deal of turbulence and uncertainty in the workplace. Work environments have altered enormously as a result of new technologies that have radically changed work practices for people in all types of organisation. Patterns of work and working hours have changed, and the pace of work has also accelerated. Competition has increased as markets have become global, and there continues to be a relentless drive for greater efficiency and increased productivity (Lisle, 1991).

In the UK and in many other European countries, there has been a large increase in the number of people working in the service industry, with a corresponding decline in those working in the manufacturing industry. In Britain, over two-thirds of those employed are now working in service industries. There has been a marked trend away from full-time male employment, with a significant increase in the number of part-time workers, particularly women, and in service industry shift work (OPCS, 1992). It is hardly surprising that job insecurity is now commonplace and that uncertainty about the future is a fact for many industries and their workforces. Even the previously secure industries such as banking and insurance have been shaken by the rapidity of change. Companies face the ever-present possibility of mergers and take-overs, no longer being able to give their employees a guarantee of a lifelong career.

A pattern of redundancy and unemployment, frequent job change and an increasing need for mobility has emerged and shows no sign of abating as the 21st century advances. Changes of this magnitude affecting the values, concepts, beliefs and norms of society have been described by Kuhn (1970) as paradigm shifts, that is, fundamental changes in the basic pattern.

The current situation requires a new health paradigm to fulfil the changing views and needs of society. There is a growing awareness of and an urgent need to place more emphasis on the environment and ecological issues. Organisations are beginning to recognise their responsibility to develop new strategies in order to address these global environmental problems. They also have an opportunity to create a different kind of workplace, which could play an important part in the development of a new approach to health.

The World Health Organization's Regional Director for Europe has pointed out that as the stability of organisations is threatened by rapidly changing markets, their ability to survive requires much more than the approaches used in the past:

> Today we require, a courageous change in attitudes, a more open, communication between workers and management and a new willingness to enter into a real dialogue and to share more seriously the responsibility for finding solutions that are acceptable both to workers and to management. (Asvall 1991: 53)

The infrastructure of the workplace is continually changing, with the current tendency to the decentralisation and fragmentation of the larger organisations. There are problems of access to the very large number of small workplaces where the labour turnover is high. Such factors present an enormous challenge for organisational health provision – how to design support and services to meet the health needs of so many different types of workforce.

The changing world of work is reflected in the Health and Safety Commission's (HSC's) Strategy Statement *Revitalising Health and Safety* (DETR, 2000), which emphasises that the health and safety system must promote a better working environment as well as preventing harm. It also focuses on occupational health as a priority. A new long-term Occupational Health Strategy has been developed by the HSC and interested parties, both within government and outside. It represents a shared agenda and joint commitment across government departments, the Scottish Executive, the National Assembly of Wales, local authorities, health authorities and a range of external stakeholders, including large and small firms, trade unions and health and other professionals. All have agreed to work in partnership to achieve challenging targets to improve occupational health in Great Britain over the next 10 years. The Occupational Health Strategy 2000 (DETR, 2000) will complement the public health strategies outlined in *Saving Lives: Our Healthier Nation* (DoH, 1999a) and other key government policies, including Welfare to Work, Sustainable Development and Modernising Government. It will have a wider view of occupational health, taking into consideration not only measures to control the effects of work on health, but also how health impinges on work and the contribution that occupational health can make to rehabilitation.

Occupational health provision

Many European countries have given a high priority to occupational health services in their general health policies. However, occupational health services in Europe vary considerably, and there are major differences between countries. In Finland, Norway, France and Germany, for example, occupational health services are a statutory part of the healthcare system, but in other countries, for example Britain, the responsibility rests with individual employers. In the UK, there is no statutory regulation requiring any occupational health service other than first aid to be provided in-house for the workforce. It tends to be the larger organisations that provide occupational health services for their employees, but only about half of the UK workforce has access to a health professional at work (Bunt, 1993).

Even for those who do have access to occupational health advice, the quantity and quality of provision varies enormously (Bamford, 1995). European models for the provision of occupational health support range from monodisciplinary, as in France, at one end of the spectrum to multi-disciplinary, as in Scandinavia, at the other. The multi-disciplinary approach offers a better model, but in some countries where occupational health provision is mandatory, links with public health remain weak. None would seem to offer a perfect model (HSC/OHAC, 2000)

In the UK, a rapidly changing pattern of employment has led to a number of perceived inequalities in occupational health. In the public sector, almost half the total workforce has access to some form of occupational health provision, but this is not the case in the private sector, where fewer than 10 per cent of organisations provide occupational health for their employees.

The National Health Service (NHS) is the largest employer in Europe, and its role as a leader in workplace health policies should be exemplary as NHS workplace health policies affect patient care. Policies must therefore ensure safe working practices, including the organisation of work, which will benefit the health of employees and hence their ability to care effectively for patients. The Clinical Governance framework offers a mechanism for improving the development of occupational health practice and service provision for all NHS employees.

Clinical Governance is a major feature of government policy, with the aim of reforming and revitalising healthcare throughout the UK (DoH, 1999b). Clinical Governance requires healthcare practitioners, including those in occupational health, to work together in a collaborative way and therefore has the potential to impact on every aspect of service delivery. The need for appropriately educated practitioners with the skills and competence to deliver care is as important within occupational health as it is in other healthcare settings (Ferguson, 2000). Standards and systems of audit within occupational health are essential. Throughout the 1990s, however, there has been a proliferation of contract occupational health service (OHS) providers, which has exacerbated the problem of setting standards. There is currently no comprehensive information available about who is delivering occupational healthcare or about where services are based.

An increasing proportion of the working population is self-employed or employed in small and medium-sized enterprises (SMEs), with little or no access to occupational health support. In the UK, SMEs account for 99 per cent of private sector businesses. Most are very small indeed, having fewer than five employees. Although the need for occupational health support is similar in both large and small organisations, each has different considerations. Small businesses have a very high turnover and a constant struggle to survive, so occupational health provision has to be cheap, convenient and particularly cost-effective (HSC/OHAC, 2000). For many workers, primary care will be the main source of advice on work-related ill health. Thus, a large part of occupational healthcare for SMEs is likely to be accessed through primary care groups (PCGs), which came into operation in 1999 and are responsible for providing primary care services for particular localities. The function of PCGs is to improve the health of their populations as well as to improve primary care locally. PCGs will aim to address occupational health issues in a various ways, for example via health improvement programmes.

Organisational health policies: a comprehensive approach

Many organisations have only minimal policies on health and safety, with no specific occupational health policy; moreover, existing guidelines on occupational health are often outdated. Much ill health at work, for example stress-related illness and musculo-skeletal disorders is multifactorial in origin, and heart disease occurs more frequently when certain working conditions prevail. Occupational health policies should, therefore, reflect the need for a holistic and integrated approach to health management. Policies should be more comprehensive to include not only health protection, but also health promotion and psychosocial issues.

So far, very little has been done to create policies to protect or promote the psychological health of the workforce. A survey of occupational health services in Europe by the World Health Organization (WHO) (1990) showed that psychological provision in the workplace was very limited, although a number of countries mentioned psychological hazards as targets for activity. A recent three-year study commissioned by the Health and Safety Executive (HSE) (Smith et al., 2000) found that stress at work was a very major problem. Some large organisations have attempted to address mental health issues, but with a tendency to focus on stress at an individual level rather than as an organisational issue.

A comprehensive approach should aim, therefore, not only to prevent injuries and illness, but also actively to promote health. Health policies need to encompass this proactive dimension. Within individual organisations, the links between the physical and mental health of the workforce must be under-stood by management. Work has become more intense throughout the 1990s, employees claiming that the pace of work has increased. At the same time, job insecurity has become more widespread, and employees are less trusting of management (Burchell et al., 1999). In order to be healthy, an organisation needs to develop health policies that address both the physical and psycholog-ical problems encountered in the workplace. The aim should be to create a work environment supportive of positive health practices based on a belief that a healthy organisation requires healthy employees. Merely urging employees to take more responsibility for their health and providing the opportunity to do so will not be effective without a supportive corporate culture.

The workplace should be a focus for the development and implementation of new health policies. The health of the working population is of vital importance to the economy as well as to the prosperity of local populations. The contemporary workplace, and its workforce, has become a crucial public health concern. Ensuring that new health policies in the workplace include both health protection and health promotion offers an opportunity to promote the health of a key sector of the population (Faculty of Public Health Medicine, 1995).

Improving health in the workplace

Working conditions have a significant influence on health status and well-being. A work-related inequality in health is prevalent in many occupational categories, for example shift workers and those in jobs with high demands and low control over their work. A recent study of nurses in the USA has shown that women in jobs with high demands, low control and low social support are at greatest risk of ill health. It also revealed that the decline in health associated with job strain is as large as that associated with smoking and a sedentary lifestyle. Current solutions target individuals rather than their social environment and tend to deal with symptoms rather than causes. These new findings have major implications for future health promotion strategies within hospitals (Cheng et al., 2000).

The workplace is therefore an important setting for preventive activities, and since people spend about one-third of their waking hours at work, the workplace has a considerable potential for health promotion. The workplace was considered to have a key role to play in achieving the four main objec-tives of *Health for All* (WHO, 1993):

- greater equity in health;
- the promotion and facilitation of a healthy lifestyle;
- a reduction in the burden of preventable ill health;
- a reorientation of the healthcare system.

It is increasingly difficult to distinguish between illness caused by work and illness arising from other causes. There are no clear boundaries, many health problems, for example cardiovascular disease, developing over a long period and having multiple causes. This broader view of occupational health allows for factors related to lifestyle, for example alcohol and drug abuse to be tackled (Schilling, 1989). The overall aim is to promote the general health of workers and their physical, mental and social well-being, as well as to optimise working conditions so that the work is better adapted to the workers in terms of both their physiological and psychological needs.

The overall aims of an organisational health strategy should be:

- to provide a safe and healthy workplace;
- to promote the optimal physical and mental health of all employees;
- to strengthen the relationship between health and productivity so that employees can contribute effectively to the organisation's goals as well as enhancing their own personal well-being.

The Canadian Government (Health Canada, 1995/99) have developed a Workplace Health System for promoting a healthy workplace, which identifies five guiding principles:

- meet the needs of all employees regardless of their current level of health.
- recognise the needs, preferences and attitudes of different groups of participants.
- recognise that an individual's lifestyle is made up of an interdependent set of health habits.
- adapt to the special features of each workplace environment.
- support the development of a strong overall health policy in the workplace.

In order to provide a safe and healthy workplace, health protection policies must cover the assessment of health risk that could cause, aggravate or contribute to ill health and that might lead to other problems, for example sickness absence. An assessment of fitness for work requires a consideration of the medical aspects of selection, job change, rehabilitation and ill health retirement, while policies on occupational disease prevention must aim to identify at-risk groups, particularly those exposed to certain hazards, either physical or psychological (Edwards et al., 1988).

Policies on health promotion should be developed alongside those on health protection. A proactive organisation will formulate specific policies on alcohol and drug abuse, smoking and the prevention of stress in relation to the management of change, as well as policies aimed at heart disease prevention and counselling for employees with problems. The national health promotion strategy *Saving Lives: Our Healthier Nation* (DoH, 1999a) identifies the workplace as one of the important settings for tackling the UK's major health problems: heart disease, mental ill health, cancer and accidents. Firmly linking occupational health with the public health strategy and increasingly aligning environmental and occupational health are important steps towards encouraging the development of healthier workplaces. A joint statement in 1999 from the Department of Health and the HSE aimed to put health into the mainstream of business life. However, although many employers acknowledge that they have an important role to play in improving employee health, they are reluctant to make a commitment to policies that appear to be remote from organisational goals.

Strategies need to be dynamic and project something positive, for example that support for employees is vital while organisations are restructuring. Such strategies will have a direct bearing on productivity and employee morale. Job satisfaction and efficiency are inseparable. An adequate standard of health and safety provision is a prerequisite for workplace health promotion. Nothing will be gained by a superficial approach; organisations need to make a genuine commitment to health, recognising that, in looking beyond immediate short-term gains, they are building a sound foundation for the future. Gaining genuine and lasting commitment is, however, likely to be the greatest challenge since the turbulence of today's global markets means that the long-term survival of any organisation is increasingly less certain.

Promoting mental health at work

A recent survey commissioned by the HSE (Smith et al., 2000) found that one in five workers suffered from a high level of stress at work, indicating that occupational stress is more prevalent than previous reports had suggested. The HSC published a discussion document, *Managing Stress at Work*, to encourage debate (HSC, 1999). The majority of respondents felt that stress at work was a serious problem and a health, safety and welfare issue, that is, that it should be dealt with by the HSC/HSE and local authorities under health and safety law. The introduction of regulatory requirements is currently under review, but in order to ensure that employers take effective action, the HSE is embarking on a wide-ranging strategy to tackle work-related stressors. This strategy is incorporated in the UK's new Occupational Health Strategy, referred to above.

In 1988, the HSE pointed out the value of instituting an occupational health policy, including a consideration of all aspects of mental health. Evidence is increasing that unsatisfactory work environments lead to psychological disorder. Karasek and Theorell (1990) have shown that it is not the demands of the work itself but the organisational structure of the work that plays the most consistent role in the development of stress-related illness. Jobs that give workers little opportunity to make decisions or to decide which skills to use are wasteful of their actual capabilities. More recently, the Whitehall II study demonstrated how the design of work affected people's mental well-being and related health outcomes (Stansfeld et al., 1999). Adverse psychosocial factors are also risk factors for cardiovascular illness, providing an explanation for the higher mortality from coronary heart disease of workers in the lower social classes, who are more likely to experience psychosocial stress at work. Policies should therefore be developed to address psychological job design and its health and productivity consequences.

Cox et al. (1990) suggest that organisational health is about more than the sum of the health of individual employees. Simply attempting to represent the health of an organisation in terms of employee health profiles (for example, blood pressure or cholesterol level) is thus inadequate. The central idea is that the organisation offers a number of different environments to employees, the qualities of which are a powerful predictor of important organisational issues such as staff turnover and absence. It can therefore be seen that policies on health need to be considered alongside policies on employment, in terms of the work environment and as an integral part of company policy. Work–life balance issues are also beginning to gain attention as employers come to recognise, for example, that an unofficial expectation that employees will routinely work long hours may not only compromise health and safety but also productivity. In other words, there is increasing evidence that effective practices to promote work–life balance will benefit the organisation as well as its employees.

Occupational health provision: services and support

An occupational health service (OHS) is responsible for providing advice concerning the health of people at work, the cost being borne by the employer. In order to be effective throughout the organisation and in order to operate in a proactive way, OHSs must have the commitment of the senior management and the board of a company. There should be corporate leadership on health to set the standards for health and communicate these to all levels of the organisation. The professional in charge of the OHS must also have access to the most senior level of management in the company, if required, and the occupational health team must be able to operate impartially at all levels of the organisation.

The OHS may include medical, nursing and occupational hygiene services as well as, when required, contributions from members of other disciplines, for example ergonomists and psychologists. The range of activities is broad, but the emphasis is on prevention rather than cure.

The main functions of a well-developed OHS (WHO, 1990) are as follows:

- surveillance of the work environment;
- initiatives and advice on the control of hazards at work;
- surveillance of the health of employees;
- follow-up of the health of vulnerable groups;

- adaptation of work and the work environment to the worker;
- organisation of first-aid and emergency responses;
- health education and health promotion;
- the collection of information on workers' health.

Although these activities have usually focused on the physical work environment, they apply equally to the psychosocial work environment and the mental health of employees. The occupational health activities listed meet the WHO and International Labour Organisation guidelines (ILO, 1985). A WHO (1990) survey of OHSs showed that the psychosocial aspects of occupational health in Europe had so far received little attention. The 1990s has seen an improvement in this respect, but the response is very uneven and it is not clear which interventions are of most value.

Relationship with employees

Employees must be able to view the OHS as a resource that they can use to resolve problems and difficulties, as well as to seek advice and guidance, in order to minimise the effect on their work performance without detriment to their jobs and career prospects. Unless the OHS is seen by employees as being impartial and confidential, it will not have any credibility with them, thus negating its usefulness as a resource. This is particularly important with regard to mental health problems (Lisle, 1991).

An OHS should, however, collaborate to help management to recognise situations that are potentially hazardous or stressful and to identify groups of employees at particular risk. Occupational health professionals should play an active role in the identification of adverse psychosocial factors and advising management on prevention and control (Schilling, 1998).

Types of occupational health provision

Good occupational health practice is one of the factors that should lead to a positive outcome for both employees and employers. Many workers in small businesses, however, are likely to remain reliant on primary care, trade unions and safety representatives for advice (HSC/OHAC, 2000). The term 'occupational health support' is used to indicate the range of advice available to SMEs.

OHSs are organised in a variety of ways and are delivered by a wide range of providers. At one end of the spectrum, provision is limited to first aid and minor treatment services provided in the workplace. Group services are independent services that provide for several workplaces in the same locality. They may, for example, serve a large number of SMEs within an industrial estate. Some firms retain local general practitioners to provide a part-time service.

Although there has recently been a decline in provision, many large organisations have an in-house OHS that can provide a wide range of facilities and services. In Scandinavia, there are specialised OHSs for specific industries, for example a nation-wide service for the Swedish construction industry.

The planning of occupational health activities must start with identifying the needs of the organisation and the specific hazards in the workplace. Further requirements of an OHS are:

- to be an impartial, advisory and expert function;
- to work on a preventive basis;
- to be staffed by personnel trained for the purpose;
- to have competence and resources for vocational rehabilitation;
- to be integrated or coordinated with the firm's health and safety committees;
- to be user friendly.

Some ways in which an OHS can assist

Assessment and diagnosis of problems

This is especially important in connection with poor work performance and the early identification of specific problems, for example alcohol dependency and stress, in individuals or groups of workers. There is a very large burden of minor mental health problems that goes largely unnoticed, since they do not result in referral to specialists, but which contribute significantly to poor work performance. The scope for health promotion in this area is enormous and has the potential to improve not only the health of an individual, but also that of the organisation as a whole.

More than 11 million working days are lost each year because of back pain, costing industry £5 billion. The HSE estimates that workplace ill health and accidents cost society up to £18 billion every year, back pain being the largest single cause of ill health at work and sickness absence. Under the umbrella of the Healthy Workplace Initiative, the Back in Work project, supported by the Trades Union Congress, the Confederation of British Industry and individual employers throughout the country, aims to tackle the problem of back pain in the workplace.

Assessment of fitness for work, and rehabilitation

The assessment of long-term health problems is especially important. Liaison with an employee's own doctor is crucial in order that the occupational health adviser can provide essential guidance for management on fitness for work and rehabilitation.

Sickness absence

The new Occupational Health Strategy aims to reduce ill health caused or exacerbated by work. Targets have been set for a 20 per cent reduction in the incidence of work-related ill health and a 30 per cent reduction in the number of days lost to work-related ill health by 2010. Everyone who is off work because of ill health or disability is to be made aware of opportunities for rehabilitation back to work as early as possible.

An OHS can analyse short- and long-term absence and provide an assessment of individuals and groups that can lead to a reduction in absence, assisting managers to understand the underlying causes.

Monitoring 'at-risk' groups

It is important to monitor the health of people employed in certain hazardous jobs, as well as groups such as shift workers. This facilitates the early identification of health problems and action to safeguard employee well-being.

Counselling

There is much scope for both reactive and proactive counselling in the workplace, for example:

- for groups of employees experiencing organisational change or exposed to other stressful events;
- for individuals with stress, alcohol or work-related problems.

An OHS can assist employees by initiating treatment and speeding up referral.

Advice on the health effects of new work practices and new technologies

An OHS has a proactive role in giving employees simple practical advice on health issues arising from new work practices and technologies, such as VDU/display screen work.

Health promotion

Workplace health promotion includes many of the traditional activities described above, but health promotion is a larger concept than is usually evident in traditional activities in that it does not differentiate between sources of threat to health that arise within the workplace and outside. Health promotion seeks to influence the health of individuals in a positive way regardless of the source of the threat to health. Wynne (1990) and Wynne and Clarkin (1992) have described examples of good practice and innovation observed in different organisations and countries. An organisation's OHS has a central role to play in stimulating interest in health promotion and ensuring the continuity of health promotion programmes.

Other benefits of occupational health services

The presence of an occupational health team can bring about an improvement in morale of a workforce, leading to greater efficiency and productivity, improved industrial relations and a positive attitude to health, which contributes to a healthy workforce.

Links with other organisations

In order to be proactive in the health promotion field, the OHS needs to form links with many outside organisations and specialist resources. The OHS should not be a service in isolation but rather the centre of a network of services that can be made accessible to the organisation and bring to it a range of different skills.

The need for proactive organisational health provision

The speed with which change is occurring in the workplace has produced a great deal of upheaval and uncertainty. In many organisations, particularly those of the rapidly growing service sector, mental health demands have escalated. Change is a challenge, a stimulus for new ideas, but it is essential for employers to understand the stressful effect that it can have on employees. Its effect is often profound, affecting the health of the organisation as a whole and its ability to function effectively. Pressure in the workplace and in the marketplace is also having a considerable impact on OHSs.

Can OHSs tackle these complex problems? For example, how relevant is the professional training to cope with mental health issues? New occupational health priorities are developing. If the needs of the changing workplace are to be met, OHSs have to provide much more now than they did a decade ago.

Organisations need a new perception of occupational health professionals and the skills they can offer. In order to tackle problems, there is a real need for the OHS to interact with the organisation it serves and to form appropriate partnerships with organisations outside the workplace. The OHS should be a dynamic resource, playing a key role in organisational strategies to help to create healthy, caring and successful organisations (Lisle, 1991).

The responsibility for improving the health of those at work falls jointly between management, trade unions, government, health professionals and all the employees. The old model of reacting to problems when they arise must be superseded by a much more proactive and dynamic approach. Preventive strategies for health, demonstrating a recognition of the connections between the physical and psychological health of the workforce, and an awareness of working conditions, including the psychosocial environment, are essential and should be part of the operating plan of every organisation.

Occupational health policy should not be drawn up in isolation but should form part of a coherent strategy for achieving optimal health, well-being and productivity. The workplace should be a focus for the development and implementation of proactive health policies, which will be instrumental in the development of healthy organisations.

References

Asvall, J.E. (1991) Viewpoint '91. Health for all in Europe: challenge for health at work. *Occupational Medicine*, **41**: 53–4.

Bamford, M. (1995) *Work and Health*. London: Chapman & Hall.

Bunt, K. (1993) *Occupational Health Provision at Work*. Health and Safety Executive, Contract Research Report No. 57. London: HMSO.

Burchell, B., Day, D., Hudson, M. and Lapido, D. (1999) *Job Insecurity and Work Intensification*. York: York Publishing.

Cheng, Y., Kawachi, I. and Coakley, E. (2000) Association between psychosocial work characteristics and health functioning in American women: prospective study. *British Medical Journal*, **320**: 1432–6.

Cox, T., Leather, P. and Cox, S. (1990) Stress, health and organisations. *Occupational Health Review*, **23**: 13–18.

Department for the Environment, Transport and the Regions (2000) *Revitalising Health and Safety*. London: HMSO.

Department of Health (1999a) *Saving Lives: Our Healthier Nation*. London: Stationery Office.

Department of Health (1999b) *Clinical Governance: Quality in the New NHS*. London: Stationery Office.

Edwards, F., McCallum, R. and Taylor, P. (eds) (1988) *Fitness for Work*. Oxford: Oxford University Press.

Faculty of Public Health Medicine (1995) Health Promotion in the Workplace, *Guidelines for Health Promotion Number 40*. London: Faculty of Public Health Medicine.

Ferguson, D. (2000) Clinical governance and occupational health. *Occupational Health Review*, **86**: 19–23.

Health Canada (1995/99) *Workplace Health System*. Ottawa: Health Canada.

Health and Safety Commission (1999) *Managing Stress at Work*. Sudbury: HSE Books.

Health and Safety Commission (2000) *Securing Health Together*. Sudbury: HSE Books.

Health and Safety Commission/Occupational Health and Advisory Commission (2000) Report and Recommendations on Improving Access to Occupational Health Support. London: HSC.

International Labour Organisation (1985) *Convention 161 and Recommendation 171 on Occupational Health Services*. London: ILO.

Karasek, R. and Theorell, T. (1990) *Healthy Work: Stress, Productivity and the Recon-struction of Working Life*. New York: Basic Books.

Kuhn, T. (1970) *The Structure of Scientific Revolutions*. Chicago: Chicago Press.

Lisle, J. (1991) Workplace transformations. In Draper, P. (ed.) *Health Through Public Policy*. London: Green Print.

Office of Population Censuses and Surveys (1992) *Labour Force Survey 1990 and 1991*. Series LFS No. 9. London: HMSO.

Schilling, R.S.F. (1989) Health protection and promotion at work. *British Journal of Industrial Medicine*, **46**(10): 683–8.

Schilling, R. (1998) *A Challenging Life*. London: Canning Press.

Smith, A., Wadsworth, E. and Johal, S. (2000) *The Scale of Occupational Stress: The Bristol Health at Work Study*. Sudbury: HSE Books.

Stansfeld, S., Head, J. and Marmot, M. (1999) *Work Related Factors and Ill-health: The Whitehall II Study*. Sudbury: HSE Books.

World Health Organization (1990) *Occupational Health Services – an Overview*. Regional Publications European Series No. 26. Copenhagen: WHO.

World Health Organization (1993) *Health for All Targets. The Health Policy for Europe* (updated edn). Copenhagen: WHO.

Wynne, R. (1990) *Innovative Workplace Actions for Health: An Overview of the Situation in Seven European Countries*. Dublin: Work Research Centre.

Wynne, R. and Clarkin, N. (1992) *European Foundation for the Improvement of Living and Working Conditions. Under Construction – Building for Health in the EC Workplace*. Luxembourg: Office for Official Publications of the European Communities.

Author Index

Subject Index